1

O A I D

OXFORD AMERICAN INFECTIOUS DISEASE LIBRARY

Healthcare Associated Infections: A Case-based Approach to Diagnosis and Management

O A I D L

OXFORD AMERICAN INFECTIOUS DISEASE LIBRARY

Healthcare Associated Infections: A Case-based Approach to Diagnosis and Management

Stephen G. Weber, MD, MS

Associate Professor, Section of Infectious Diseases and Global Health
Chief Medical Officer and Vice President for Clinical Effectiveness
University of Chicago Medicine
Chicago, IL

Cassandra D. Salgado, MD, MS

Associate Professor, Division of Infectious Diseases
Medical Director of Infection Control
Medical University of South Carolina
Charleston, SC

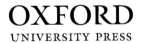

OXFORD
UNIVERSITY PRESS

OXFORD
UNIVERSITY PRESS

Oxford University Press is a department of the University of Oxford.
It furthers the University's objective of excellence in research, scholarship,
and education by publishing worldwide.

Oxford   New York

Auckland   Cape Town   Dar es Salaam   Hong Kong   Karachi
Kuala Lumpur   Madrid   Melbourne   Mexico City   Nairobi
New Delhi   Shanghai   Taipei   Toronto

With offices in

Argentina   Austria   Brazil   Chile   Czech Republic   France   Greece
Guatemala   Hungary   Italy   Japan   Poland   Portugal   Singapore
South Korea   Switzerland   Thailand   Turkey   Ukraine   Vietnam

Oxford is a registered trademark of Oxford University Press in the UK
and certain other countries.

Published in the United States of America by
Oxford University Press
198 Madison Avenue, New York, NY 10016

© Oxford University Press 2013

Library of Congress Cataloging-in-Publication Data

Healthcare associated infections : a case-based approach to diagnosis and management /
[edited by] Stephen G. Weber, Cassandra Salgado.
p. ; cm. — (Oxford American infectious disease library)
Includes bibliographical references and index.
ISBN 978-0-19-979638-0 (hardback : alk. paper)
I. Weber, Stephen G.   II. Salgado, Cassandra.   III. Series: Oxford American infectious
disease library.
[DNLM: 1. Cross Infection—diagnosis.   2. Cross Infection—prevention &
control.   3. Infection Control—methods. WX 167]
616.9'11—dc23   2012016022

9 8 7 6 5 4 3 2
Printed in the United States of America
on acid-free paper

Dedicated to my family, mentors, and students and all those who have dedicated themselves to preventing and curing infection.

—Stephen Weber

Dedicated to my providers at the Medical University of South Carolina whose thoughtful expertise and care kept me in good health through completion of this project and to my partner who supports all of my academic endeavors.

—Cassandra Salgado

Contents

Contributors

Natasha Bagdasarian, MD, MPH
University of Michigan Health System,
Department of Internal Medicine
Divisions of General Medicine and
Infectious Diseases
Veteran Affairs Ann Arbor Health
System
Ann Arbor, MI

David B. Banach, MD, MPH
Division of Infectious Diseases
Weill Cornell Medical College
New York, NY

Maureen Bolon, MD, MS
Associate Professor of Medicine
Medical Director of Infection Control
and Prevention
Northwestern Memorial Hospital
Chicago, IL

Meghan Brennan, MD
University of Wisconsin School of
Medicine and Public Health
Madison, WI

David P. Calfee, MD, MS
Chief Hospital Epidemiologist
New York-Presbyterian Hospital/
Weill-Cornell
Associate Professor of Medicine and
Public Health
Division of Infectious Diseases
Weill Cornell Medical College
New York, NY

L.W. Preston Church, MD
Hospital Epidemiologist
Ralph H. Johnson VA
Charleston, SC

Christopher J. Crnich, MD, MS
University of Wisconsin School of
Medicine and Public Health
William S. Middleton Veterans
Administration Hospital
Madison, WI

Curtis J. Coley II, MD
Division of Pulmonary and Critical Care
University of Michigan
Ann Arbor, MI

Sara Cosgrove, MD, MS
Associate Professor of Medicine,
Division of Infectious Diseases
Director, Antimicrobial Stewardship
Program
Associate Hospital Epidemiologist
Johns Hopkins Medical Institutions
Baltimore, MD

Daniel Diekema, MD
Division of Infectious Diseases
Department of Internal Medicine
University of Iowa Carver College of
Medicine
Iowa City, IA

Terry C. Dixon, MD, PhD
Division of Pediatric Infectious
Diseases
Department of Pediatrics
Medical University of South Carolina
Charleston, SC

**Jennifer C. Esbenshade,
MD, MPH**
Vanderbilt University School of
Medicine
Department of Pediatrics, Division of
Hospital Medicine
Nashville, TN

Charlesnika T. Evans, PhD, MPH
Center for Management of Complex
Chronic Care
Edward Hines Jr. Department of
Veterans Affairs Hospital
Hines, IL
Institute for Healthcare Studies
Northwestern University
Transplant Outcomes Collaborative
(NUTORC)
Feinberg School of Medicine,
Northwestern University
Chicago, IL

Sandra Fowler, MD, MSc
Associate Professor of Pediatrics
Director, Division of Pediatric
Infectious Diseases
Medical University of South Carolina
Charleston, SC

Melanie Gerrior, MD
Division of Infectious Diseases
Medical University of
South Carolina
Charleston, SC

Keith W. Hamilton, MD
University of Pennsylvania School of
Medicine
Philadelphia, PA

Courtney Hebert, MD
Post-Doctoral Researcher
Department of Biomedical Informatics
Clinical Assistant Professor
Division of Infectious Diseases
The Ohio State University Wexner
Medical Center
Columbus, OH

Michael Heung, MD, MS
University of Michigan Health
System, Department of Internal
Medicine
Division of Nephrology
Ann Arbor, MI

Aimee Hodowanec, MD
Rush University Medical Center and
Stroger Hospital of Cook County
Chicago, IL

Michael G. Ison, MD, MS
Divisions of Infectious Diseases and
Organ Transplantation
Northwestern University
Comprehensive Transplant Center
Feinberg School of Medicine,
Northwestern University
Chicago, IL

Evgenia Kagan, MD
Assistant Professor of Medicine
Division of Infectious Diseases
Medical University of South Carolina
Charleston, SC

Keith Kaye, MD
Division of Infectious Diseases
Wayne State University
Detroit, MI

J. Michael Kilby, MD
Professor of Medicine and
Microbiology/Immunology
Director, Division of Infectious
Diseases
Medical University of South Carolina
Charleston, SC

**Ebbing Lautenbach, MD, MPH,
MSCE**
Associate Professor of Medicine and
Epidemiology
Senior Scholar, Center for Clinical
Epidemiology and Biostatistics
Associate Director, Clinical Epidemio-
logy Unit (Educational Programs)
Director of Research, Department
of Healthcare Epidemiology and
Infection Control
University of Pennsylvania School of
Medicine
Philadelphia, PA

Michael Y. Lin, MD, MPH
Section of Infectious Diseases
Rush University Medical Center
Chicago, IL

Preeti N. Malani, MD, MSJ
Divisions of Geriatric Medicine and
Infectious Diseases
Veteran Affairs Ann Arbor Health
System
Geriatric Research Education and
Clinical Center (GRECC)
Ann Arbor, MI

Dror Marchaim, MD
Division of Infectious Diseases
Wayne State University
Detroit, MI

Camelia Marculescu, MD, MSCR
Associate Professor of Medicine
Division of Infectious Diseases
Medical University of South Carolina
Charleston, SC

Melissa A. Miller, MD, MS
Division of Pulmonary & Critical
Care Medicine
University of Michigan
Ann Arbor, MI

Sarah Miller, MD
Division of Infectious Diseases
Johns Hopkins School of Medicine
Baltimore, MD

Rebekah Moehring, MD
Duke University Medical Center,
Division of Infectious Diseases
Durham, NC

Carlene A. Muto, MD, MS
Associate Professor of Medicine and
Epidemiology
Division of Hospital Epidemiology
and Infection Control,
University of Pittsburgh Medical
Center, Presbyterian Campus
Pittsburgh, PA

Shephali H. Patel, DO
Section of Infectious Diseases
Rush University Medical Center
Chicago, IL

Kyle J. Popovich, MD
Rush University Medical Center and
Stroger Hospital of Cook County
Chicago, IL

Ari Robicsek, MD
University of Chicago Pritzker School
of Medicine
Chicago, IL
Departments of Medicine and
Medical Informatics
NorthShore University HealthSystem
Evanston, IL

Andrew T. Root, MD
Northwestern University Feinberg
School of Medicine
Division of Infectious Disease
Chicago, IL

Cassandra D. Salgado, MD, MS
Associate Professor, Division of
Infectious Diseases
Medical Director of Infection
Control
Medical University of South Carolina
Charleston, SC

Michael J. Satlin, MD
Weill Cornell Medical College
New York, NY

Pranavi Sreeramoju, MD, MPH
Department of Medicine-Infectious
Diseases
University of Texas Southwestern
Medical Center
Dallas, TX

Jeremy C. Storm, DO
Infectious Diseases
Infectious Disease Specialists
Sioux Falls, SD

Thomas R. Talbot, MD, MPH
Vanderbilt University School of
Medicine
Department of Medicine, Division of
Infectious Diseases
Nashville, TN

Nicole Theodoropoulos, MD
Divisions of Infectious Diseases and
Organ Transplantation
Northwestern University
Comprehensive Transplant Center
Northwestern University Feinberg
School of Medicine
Chicago, IL

Stephen G. Weber, MD, MS
Associate Professor, Section of
Infectious Diseases and Global Health
Chief Medical Officer and Vice
President for Clinical Effectiveness
University of Chicago Medicine
Chicago, IL

Sharon B. Wright, MD
Silverman Institute for Healthcare
Quality and Division of Infectious
Diseases
Beth Israel Deaconess Medical
Center
Boston, MA

David S. Yassa, MD
Silverman Institute for Healthcare
Quality and Division of Infectious
Diseases
Beth Israel Deaconess Medical
Center
Boston, MA

**Teresa R. Zembower,
MD, MPH**
Northwestern University Feinberg
School of Medicine
Division of Infectious Disease
Chicago, IL

Disclosure statements

Natasha Bagdasarian has nothing to disclose.

David B. Banach has nothing to disclose.

Maureen Bolon has nothing to disclose.

Meghan Brennan has nothing to disclose.

David P. Calfee received research support from the Association of American Medical Colleges.

L.W. Preston Church is a speaker for "The Faces of Flu," a program sponsored by Rush University with support via unrestricted educational grants from Gilead and Genentech.

Christopher J. Crnich has received research support from the University of Wisconsin CTSA and the Hartford Center for Excellence.

Curtis J. Coley II has nothing to disclose.

Sara Cosgrove has nothing to disclose.

Daniel Diekema has received research support from Merck, Pfizer, Innovative Biosensors, bioMerieux, Cerexa, and PurThread Technologies.

Terry C. Dixon has nothing to disclose.

Jennifer C. Esbenshade has received research support from MedImmune.

Charlesnika T. Evans has received research funding from Merck.

Sandra Fowler has nothing to disclose.

Melanie Gerrior has nothing to disclose.

Keith W. Hamilton has nothing to disclose.

Courtney Hebert has nothing to disclose.

Michael Heung has nothing to disclose.

Aimee Hodowanec has nothing to disclose.

Michael G. Ison has received research support from BioCryst, Chimerix, GlaxoSmithKlein, Roche, and ViraCor; has been a paid consultant for Crucell and Toyama/MediVector; has been an unpaid consultant for BioCryst, Biota, Cellex, Clarassance, GlaxoSmithKlein, MP Bioscience, NexBio, Genentech/ Roche, Toyama, and T2 Diagnostics; and has been on data and safety monitoring boards for Chimerix and NexBio.

Evgenia Kagan has nothing to disclose.

Keith Kaye has received honoraria from Cubist and has served a consultant for Merck, Pfizer, and Theradoc.

J. Michael Kilby has nothing to disclose.

Ebbing Lautenbach has nothing to disclose.

Michael Y. Lin has nothing to disclose.

Preeti N. Malani has nothing to disclose.

Dror Marchaim has nothing to disclose.

Camelia Marculescu has nothing to disclose.

Melissa A. Miller has received research support from an NIH/NHLBI training grant.

Sarah Miller has nothing to disclose.

Rebekah Moehring has nothing to disclose.

Carlene A. Muto was on a speaker bureau for Robert Michael Educational Institute LLC.

Kyle J Popovich has nothing to disclose.

Ari Robicsek has nothing to disclose.

Andrew T. Root has nothing to disclose.

Cassandra D. Salgado has received research funding from the Department of defense and AHRQ.

Michael J. Satlin has nothing to disclose.

Pranavi Sreeramoju has nothing to disclose.

Jeremy Storm has nothing to disclose.

Thomas R. Talbot received research support from Sanofi Pasteur and has served a consultant for Joint Community Resources, Community Health Systems.

Nicole Theodoropoulos has nothing to disclose.

Stephen G. Weber has consulted for Joint Commission Resources.

Sharon B. Wright was a speaker and developer for the SHEA/CDC Healthcare-Associated Infections Course.

Shephali H. Patel has nothing to disclose.

David S. Yassa has nothing to disclose.

Teresa R. Zembower has nothing to disclose.

Chapter 1a

Approach to the Management of Patients with Suspected Healthcare-Associated Infection

Cassandra D. Salgado and Stephen G. Weber

Introduction

Despite recent advances, healthcare-associated infections (HAI) pose continued diagnostic and therapeutic challenges to even well-trained and experienced clinicians. In this book, dozens of cases of frequently encountered HAI are introduced and discussed by some of the most dynamic and expert clinicians in the fields of Healthcare Epidemiology, Infection Prevention, and Infectious Diseases. In each case, a comprehensive overview of the diagnosis and subsequent treatment of a patient or patients affected by HAI is described. In addition, key strategies and practices for the prevention of HAI are introduced.

In order to set the stage for this comprehensive discussion of specific clinical scenarios, it is useful to first provide an overview of the general approach to the management of affected patients. The principles described in this first introductory chapter will provide the reader with a broad understanding of the unique challenges to the diagnosis and initial treatment of HAI. The structured approach outlined here, when applied consistently at the bedside, can help to ensure that even the most complex and challenging HAI is managed in a timely, appropriate, and evidence-based manner.

In the following chapter, the principles and practices of hospital-based infection prevention are introduced. The rigorous conduct of infectious diseases surveillance, performance improvement, and outbreak investigation largely remain the responsibility of dedicated specialists in infection prevention and healthcare epidemiology. However, the critical role of every provider in preventing infection, including physicians, nurses, and other care professionals, has become increasingly apparent as the incidence of HAI increases and demands for control and elimination mount. With the introduction provided in chapter 1b, the reader should be better equipped to meet this important responsibility.

Microbiology and Pathogenesis

In general, there are two principle factors that contribute to the increased risk of serious infection among patients in healthcare facilities. First, when compared to the commensal bacteria with which healthy hosts are generally colonized, the spectrum of microbes to which patients are exposed in hospitals, long-term care facilities, and other clinical settings are often more virulent and more resistant to common antimicrobial therapy. Particularly in the acute care setting, patients are exposed to antibiotics and other therapies that have the consequence of eradicating or at least modifying the diversity of harmless (and often beneficial) bacteria that populate the skin, intestines, oropharynx, and other mucosal surfaces. As a result, hospitalized patients are susceptible to the acquisition of more aggressive bacterial species that are commonly encountered in this setting. For example, after even a brief hospital stay, the normal flora of the oral cavity of older patients are typically replaced by enteric gram-negative pathogens such as *E. coli* and *K. pneumoniae*. Acquisition generally comes about as a result of the horizontal transmission of such pathogens between patients, most commonly on the uncleansed hands of healthcare providers or via fomites such as shared medical equipment. To the extent that humans are most commonly infected with the same microbial organisms with which they are colonized, the replacement of the normal flora with these more virulent strains can serve as a prelude to subsequent infection.

The second main contributor to the high frequency of HAI is the compromise of the normal host defenses that occurs among patients as a result of illness and even appropriate clinical care. Under the right circumstances, even less aggressive microbes can breach the normal physical and immunological barriers that typically protect the host. These breakdowns can include compromise of the integument (such as a vascular access catheter or a surgical wound), nutritional deficiencies (frequently resulting from gastrointestinal pathology or inadequate supplementation in a severely ill patient), and even frank disruptions of humeral or cellular immunity after cancer chemotherapy. In all such cases, even transient exposure to relatively less aggressive pathogens (such as coagulase-negative strains of *Staphylococcus*) can result in complicated and potentially lethal infection.

General Approach to Management

In light of this understanding of the pathogenesis of HAI, an appreciation of local microbial epidemiology and individual patient risk factors is essential to the appropriate management of these infections. More specifically, the optimal approach to initial diagnosis and treatment of the patient with known or suspected HAI can be distilled down to a handful of principles. These are illustrated in Figure 1.1 and described in greater detail in the sections that follow.

Identify the Causative Pathogen

The first step to managing a patient with known or suspected HAI is to identify the probable causative pathogen. Initially, the treating clinician should seek to

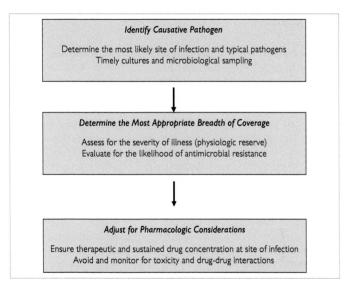

Figure 1.1 General approach to the management of the patient with known or suspected healthcare-associated infection.

determine the most likely body site of infection. In making this assessment, the astute clinician must be prepared to examine the patient carefully for subtle signs and symptoms. Such attention to detail should be sustained throughout hospitalization; a part of the daily routine for the clinician responsible for the care of high-risk patients. A few simple observations at the bedside can be extremely helpful in determining whether HAI is developing, or when one is suspected to quickly discern the most likely site of infection. Key elements of such an evaluation include assessment of surgical wounds and other skin breaks for signs of inflammation. Given the frequency of infection involving intravascular catheters, careful inspection and palpation of such sites for warmth, tenderness, or erythema is crucial and must be incorporated into even the most cursory bedside physical exam. A thorough lung and abdominal exam are also important to help exclude common HAI at these sites.

Having determined the probable site of infection, the knowledgeable clinician should be able to predict the most likely causative pathogen based on personal experience and the published medical literature (Table 1.1). For example, most will be aware that bloodstream infections associated with central venous lines are most commonly caused by coagulase negative staphylococci, *Staphylococcus aureus* and *Candida* spp. Such general knowledge should be supplemented by appreciation of the local epidemiology of HAI. For example, the physician may be aware that gram-negative pathogens have recently been the cause of a large number of central line-associated bloodstream infections at the hospital and may adjust her initial recommendation for empirical therapy accordingly.

Table 1.1 Bacterial pathogens typically associated with healthcare-associated infection at various body sites

Body Site/ Infection	Most Common Causative Pathogens	Other Associated Pathogens
Skin/Wound	*Staphylococcus aureus* (MRSA) *Streptococcus spp.*	*Enterobacteriaceae* *Pseudomonas aeruginosa*
Bloodstream	Coagulase-negative *Staphylococci* *Staphylococcus aureus* (MRSA) *Candida spp.* *Enterococcus spp.*	*Pseudomonas aeruginosa* *Enterobacteriaceae*
Lung/Pneumonia	*Pseudomonas aeruginosa* *Staphylococcus aureus* (MRSA) *Escherichia coli* *Klebsiella spp.*	*Candida spp.*
Urine	*Escherichia coli* *Klebsiella spp.* *Pseudomonas aeruginosa*	*Candida spp.* *Staphylococcus aureus* (MRSA) *Enterococcus spp.*

Of course, the definitive means by which to determine the causative pathogen is through the collection of specimens for culture and other microbiological sampling. Whenever possible, microbiological samples should be obtained before the administration of broad-spectrum antimicrobial therapy. Blood cultures are likely to be a part of virtually any workup for HAI—not only because of the high rate of primary bloodstream infections among hospitalized patients, but because so many HAI can be complicated by secondary bacteremia. In contrast, the routine collection of urinary samples may not be warranted, especially in cases in which signs and symptoms point to primary infection at another site. This raises an important general principle in interpreting the results of microbial sampling of hospitalized patients. Specifically, to conclude that a positive urine culture is necessarily indicative of serious infection in a hospitalized patient, especially in the absence of localizing signs or symptoms, is fraught with serious consequences. Clinicians run the risk of inappropriately attributing signs of infection to the urinary tract and therefore may miss the opportunity to confirm a more accurate diagnosis of infection at a different site. Indeed, the results of cultures obtained from typically unsterile sites must be interpreted extremely carefully in order to not be misled by the detection of colonizing strains, especially in the case of patients who have already been exposed to broad-spectrum antimicrobial therapy. In this circumstance, it is possible that highly resistant pathogens will be recovered from sites such as wounds, tracheal aspirates, or sputum, irrespective of whether these organisms are contributing to active infection. The end result in all such cases may be inappropriate and potentially unnecessary antibiotic treatment.

Determine the Most Appropriate Breadth of Coverage

Having established the most likely causative pathogen for HAI, the next step, even while awaiting the results of microbiological sampling, is to determine the most appropriate breadth of initial empirical therapy. In general, this decision can be reached by assessing two principle factors, the severity of the patient's clinical presentation and status as well as the likelihood of antimicrobial resistance.

The severity of illness, especially for a patient already in the intensive care unit or at high risk for hemodynamic or respiratory compromise, should significantly influence the selection of initial antimicrobial therapy by the treating clinician. Put simply, the more severely ill the patient, the greater the need for initial broad-spectrum antimicrobial coverage. In this circumstance, the treating clinician cannot afford to be wrong in choosing initial medical therapy. Were he or she to select too narrow an antimicrobial regimen, evolving infection could go effectively untreated and the patient may suffer dire consequences in terms of morbidity and even mortality. For example, a postoperative transplant patient who experiences the abrupt onset of high fever, hypotension, and end organ dysfunction should be prescribed an intensive regimen of antimicrobial therapy to include coverage for *Staphylococcus aureus*, *Pseudomonas aeruginosa*, and other gram-negative pathogens. Any one (or more) of these common pathogens can be associated with sepsis syndrome in a vulnerable hospitalized patient. In the absence of directed therapy, any of these microbes could kill the patient even before final culture results are available. In contrast, for a patient without underlying immunosuppression, even with signs of a serious infection, a more narrow approach to coverage is more sensible in that failure to cover the primary pathogen may not be associated with such dire circumstances and the selection of more narrow coverage may spare the patient the toxicity and overall risk of broad-spectrum antimicrobial coverage.

The other factor that determines the most appropriate breadth of coverage for HAI is the likelihood of antimicrobial resistance, especially in light of the continued emergence of progressively more resistant pathogens as a cause of HAI (Table 1.2). Once again, in this case, the clinician must rely on her or his knowledge of epidemiology, and particularly the impact of local trends in antimicrobial resistance. For this, the clinician depends on resources such as the hospital antimicrobial susceptibility report (antibiogram) and alerts from the hospital's Infection Prevention Department or the Public Health Department about recent outbreaks and patterns of emerging resistance. For example, the approach to the patient with a surgical wound infection is apt to be quite different for a patient infected at a facility where methicillin-resistant *Staphylococcus aureus* is rare versus one seen at a hospital where resistance is endemic. Such general data should be supplemented by knowledge of the individual patient's risk for carriage or infection with multidrug-resistant organisms (MDROs). Typical risk factors include extended hospitalization, prior antimicrobial therapy, and immunocompromised state (Table 1.3). The greater the likelihood of resistance, the broader the empiric antimicrobial coverage needed.

Adjust for Pharmacological Considerations

The final, but certainly not least important, consideration in selecting the initial empiric therapy for the patient with known or suspected HAI relates to pharmacological issues regarding the available antimicrobial agents and the affected patient. The limits of this book do not permit an in-depth discussion of

Table 1.2 Emerging multi-drug resistant organisms and typical options for antimicrobial therapy

Resistant Pathogen	Typical Options for Antimicrobial Therapy
Methicillin-resistant *Staphylococcus aureus* (MRSA)	Daptomycin
	Linezolid
	Ceftobiprole
Vancomycin-resistant *Enterococcus* (VRE)	Daptomycin
	Linezolid
	Quinupristin/Dalfopristin
Extended-spectrum beta-lactamase (ESBL) producing Enterobacteriaceae	Carbapenems (e.g. imipenem, meropenem)
	Aminoglycosides (e.g. amikacin)
	Colistin (colistimethate sodium)
Carbapenem-resistant Enterobacteriaceae (CRE)	Colistin (colistimethate sodium)
Fluconazole-resistant *Candida spp.*	Echinocandins (e.g. micafungin)

Table 1.3 Risk factors for multi-drug resistant organisms (MDRO) among hospitalized patients

MDRO Risk Factors
Exposure to systemic antimicrobial therapy
Previous or prolonged hospitalization
Comorbid medical conditions (e.g. diabetes)
Older age
Abdominal surgery
Intensive care unit stay
Immune suppression
Inadequate infection control practices

the multitude of pharmacokinetic and pharmacodynamic factors that influence this decision-making. Suffice to say that consideration must be given to ensure that the antimicrobial agent that is administered will be able to reach effective levels at the site of known or suspected infection. Proper dose adjustment and optimal timing are essential. In addition, strong consideration should be given to the principle of source control. This refers to all interventions aimed at removing or reducing (whenever possible) the primary site of infection in order to maximize the likelihood that host immunity and antimicrobial therapy will together result in clinical cure. Ultimately, the optimal management of many HAI is as much dependent on the drainage of a sequestered collection or removal of an infected prosthetic device as it is on selecting the appropriate antimicrobial agent.

When incorporating complex pharmacological considerations to the management of a patient with HAI, even the best clinicians sometimes overlook more basic aspects of the selection of appropriate antibiotic therapy. Specifically, drug hypersensitivity, toxicity, and drug interactions are especially important in managing these infections. Hospitalized patients commonly receive multiple oral and parenteral therapies to manage not only their acute illness but also their underlying comorbid conditions. Each agent is associated with its own risk of toxicity and interactions. To not consider the potential risk associated with the selection of an antimicrobial drug in this context is to run the risk of serious harm, and even death.

Suggested Reading

El-Solh AA, Pietrantoni C, Bhat A, et al. Colonization of dental plaques: a reservoir of respiratory pathogens for hospital-acquired pneumonia in institutionalized elders. Chest 2004;126:1575–1582.

Muto CA, Jernigan JA, Ostrowsky BE, et al. The Society for Healthcare Epidemiology of America guideline for preventing nosocomial transmission of multidrug-resistant strains of Staphylococcus aureus and Enterococcus. Infect Control Hosp Epidemiol 2003;24:362.

National Nosocomial Infections Surveillance (NNIS) System Report, data summary from January 1992 through June 2004, issued October 2004. Am J Infect Control 2004;32(8):470–485.

Siegel JD, Rhinehart E, Jackson M, Chiarello L, and the Healthcare Infection Control Practices Advisory Committee. Management of multidrug-resistant organisms in healthcare settings 2006. Centers for Disease Control. Available at: www.cdc.gov/ncidod/dhqp/pdf/ar/mdroGuideline2006.pdf (accessed October 7, 2011).

Chapter 1b

Overview of Hospital-Based Infection Prevention

Stephen G. Weber and Cassandra D. Salgado

Introduction

There is increasing evidence that the majority of healthcare-associated infections (HAI) are preventable. Generally, the measures that have been shown to reduce the risk of infection are conceptually simple, technically uncomplicated and dependent only on strict adherence to basic practices on the part of bedside clinicians. Unfortunately, compliance with measures such as hand hygiene and the use of personal protective equipment remains well below 100% at most centers. With this in mind, the accountability to prevent HAI does not rest entirely with those who are primarily charged with the task, and specifically those working in hospital infection control programs. Rather, every provider who has contact with patients and the hospital environment bears an important individual responsibility for the prevention of infection.

Although for the most part this book focuses on the diagnosis and management of HAI once signs and symptoms have developed, the reader will also be introduced to the practical and routine steps that can be taken at the bedside to prevent infection or at least to mitigate the risk of harm to patients. Most of the case discussions that follow include at least a brief overview of the strategies that have been demonstrated to prevent the various infections that are discussed. However, to more broadly introduce the topic of infection prevention, this chapter familiarizes the reader with the general principles that guide most infection control strategies and measures.

The chapter begins with an overview of hospital-based infection control programs. In a subsequent section, general principles of control are introduced, with an emphasis on transmission control (including environmental interventions) and strategies to protect the host from deep infection. In each case, emphasis is placed on the responsibilities of bedside providers in the prevention of infection.

Hospital Based Infection Control Programs

Personnel

Hospital-based infection prevention and control programs have established the paradigm for governance, administration, and clinical approach to the prevention of HAI across all healthcare settings (Fig. 1.2). The typical hospital-based

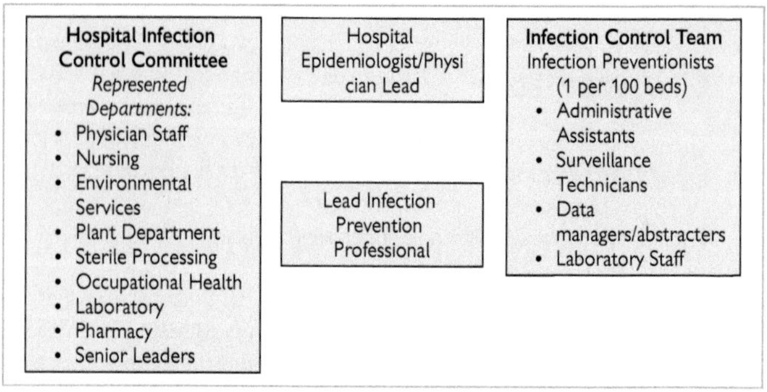

Figure 1.2 Structural elements of a typical hospital-based infection control program

infection prevention and control team includes clinically-oriented individuals with diverse backgrounds, expertise, and skill sets. Infection preventionists (IPs; a.k.a. infection control professionals or practitioners) are principally responsible for the day-to-day operations of most programs. Infection preventionists routinely engage in surveillance, performance improvement, educational activities, and outbreak investigations. Professional certification for these is available and is an increasingly expected qualification in most settings. The work of IPs may be supported by data analysts, surveillance technicians, and administrative assistants.

The engagement and contribution of the physician lead of a hospital-based infection prevention and control program may be surprisingly variable. In well-resourced settings, the physician leader often has specific training and experience in infection prevention and healthcare epidemiology. In these organizations, the physician lead is often intimately involved in setting the strategic vision of the program, establishing goals and performance measures, and spearheading performance improvement initiatives and investigations. At other organizations, the physician lead may have no specific background or training in infection prevention. He or she might only chair the institution's infection control committee and serve as a liaison with the medical staff when interventions are required.

In most hospitals, the infection control committee oversees the activities of the infection control program and serves the additional role of communicating the findings and recommendations of the program to other providers, staff and leaders at the hospital. The infection control committee is generally multidisciplinary in composition, with representatives from not only the largest clinical areas, but also hospital leadership, clinical laboratory, pharmacy, environmental services, performance improvement, regulatory compliance, and occupational medicine, to name just a few.

Activities

One of the most important responsibilities of the infection prevention and control team is to ensure that the resources and expertise of the program are deployed in such a manner to ensure that the maximal number of infections are prevented and the greatest number of patients are protected. **The infection control risk assessment**, a standardized exercise mandated by accreditation agencies such as the Joint Commission, offers a systematic approach to this practice. No less frequently than annually, the infection control team should convene with key stakeholders from around the hospital to prioritize the infectious risks facing patients, visitors, and staff. A number of tools have been developed to ensure that this work is undertaken in a quantitative and objective manner (Table 1.4).

Surveillance, the systematic collection and analysis of laboratory and clinical data to detect trends in the frequency of hospital-acquired infection and/or that of epidemiologically important organisms, is fundamental to the practice of infection control and is intimately connected to all other program activities. Typical targets for surveillance include the frequency of specific device-related infections (such as central-line associated bloodstream infections and ventilator associated pneumonia), infection or colonization with multidrug-resistant organisms (MDROs), surgical site infections, and hospital-acquired cases of seasonal influenza. Surveillance data are typically reported to both hospital leadership and frontline staff in a periodic standardized report (Table 1.5).

Through **performance improvement** activities, the infection prevention and control team undertakes local or hospital-wide programs to reduce the ongoing risk of specific infections, to interrupt the propagation of an outbreak or cluster of infections, to enhance readiness for or response to accreditation and regulatory standards, or simply to promote best practices and an overall culture of safety. The tools employed by an effective program are shared with other experts in healthcare performance improvement and quality. Increasingly,

Table 1.4 Sample Risk Assessment Tool for Hospital-Based Infection Control Program*				
Pathogen/Syndrome	Severity	Population at Risk	Vulnerability	Total Risk Score
	(1–5)	(1–5)	(1–5)	
Bloodstream infection	4	3	4	48
Surgical site Infection	3	4	4	48
MRSA	3	4	3	36
C. difficile	4	4	2	32
Influenza	2	4	3	24
Ventilator-associated infection	4	2	3	24
Resistant GNR	5	2	1	10
Urinary tract infection	1	3	3	9
Vancomycin-resistant enterococci	1	2	3	6

* In this example, a number of clinical syndromes and infections are scored according to the severity of the infection, the size of the population at risk and the likelihood that the program is prepared to manage this problem (more prepared = lower score). The severity of the risk is determined by multiplying the scores to arrive at a total risk score.

Table 1.5 Sample Report Card for Summarizing the Results of Surveillance for HAI*

Pathogen/Syndrome (number of cases)	Prior Year	Target	Year to Date	Q1	Q2	Q3	Q4
CLABSI (per 1,000 catheter days)	2.1	1.0	1.3	1.9	0.9	1.0	
Surgical Site Infection	19	13	7	3	3	1	
MRSA	30	20	17	8	5	4	
C. difficile	26	17	9	6	2	1	
Influenza	9	6	8	4	3	1	
Ventilator-associated Pneumonia	6	4	1	1	0	0	
Resistant GNR	8	5	6	2	2	2	
Urinary Tract Infection	21	14	12	6	4	2	
Vancomycin-resistant Enterococci	8	5	3	2	1	0	

*In this example, data for a number of common infections are provided on a quarterly basis (through the third quarter). A target representing a 33% reduction from the total number of each infection during the prior year has been established. Color coding could be done to indicate whether the target has been met (green) or not (red) during each reporting period.
CLABSI, central line-associated bloodstream infection.

Table 1.6 Elements of a Typical Outbreak Investigation as Conducted By a Hospital-Based Infection Control Program

Detect increase from baseline incidence
Establish preliminary case definition
Deploy immediate remediation measures
Surveillance for additional cases
Report to public health department if required
Refine case definition
Environmental examination/sampling
Structured analysis (case control study)
Deploy remediation steps

these approaches have been influenced by the application of techniques applied from other settings and industries, such as Lean and Six Sigma tools.

Outbreak investigation is perhaps the most well-known but among the least understood aspects of routine hospital-based infection prevention and control. Whether prompted by the results of surveillance data, the experience and observations of bedside clinicians, or the suspicions of an experienced IP, clusters of infection warrant timely evaluation, assessment, analysis, and intervention. In contrast to the more unstructured approach promulgated in popular fiction, outbreak investigation in the modern hospital is primarily driven by the meticulous (and sometimes tedious) review of data, thorough environmental assessments, and extensive interviews and discussions with providers and other stakeholders. Typical outbreak investigation activities are described in Table 1.6.

Regulatory compliance is another responsibility that the infection prevention and control team shares with numerous other hospital stakeholders. Accreditation bodies such as the Joint Commission, state and local boards of health, and insurance payers have developed increasingly high standards for hospital care. Although the ultimate consumer, the patient, stands to benefit from well-reasoned and evidence-based standards, to the IP and his or her colleagues, ensuring continuous compliance with these expectations can place considerable strain on even well-resourced programs.

Infection Control Principles and Strategies

General Principles

The pathogenesis and microbiological basis for healthcare-associated infection have already been introduced. With this foundation, the general approach to infection prevention can be thought of as the interplay of two distinct strategies. First is the prevention of the transmission of pathogenic microbes from one patient to others through the use of a variety of physical, chemical, and environmental barriers. The second approach is to mitigate the risk that patients exposed to such pathogens will become infected as a result of the compromise of host defenses. These two activities are described in the sections that follow and are summarized in Table 1.7.

A parallel activity in the prevention of infection, and especially those caused by MDROs, is antimicrobial stewardship. Without question, antibiotic use, misuse, and abuse are primarily responsible for the proliferation of increasingly resistant and virulent pathogens, including carbapenem-resistant gram negatives, methicillin-resistant *Staphylococcus aureus*, and *Clostridium difficile*. Therefore, the judicious use of antimicrobial therapy in all healthcare settings has the potential for supporting the work of transmission control and host protection. The medical literature describes the favorable impact of multiple stewardship interventions, including drug restriction, postprescription review and optimization of periprocedural antimicrobial prophylaxis. A complete description and review of antimicrobial stewardship is beyond the scope of this text and the reader is referred to more comprehensive and authoritative reviews of the subject.

Table 1.7 General Principles of Hospital Based Infection Prevention

Transmission Control	Mitigation Against Serious Infection
Hand hygiene	CLABSI Prevention Bundle
Personal protective equipment	Head of bed elevation (VAP)
Instrument decontamination & sterilization	Perioperative antibiotic prophylaxis (SSI)
Environmental decontamination	Mupirocin nasal eradication (MRSA)
	Perioperative glycemic control
	Chlorhexidine skin preparation/bathing

Barrier Precautions to Transmission

The principle measures to reduce the risk of nearly all HAI remain the barriers that can be established between patients. **Hand hygiene** serves as the prototypical application of this approach. Although increased adherence to hand hygiene standards has been associated with significant decreases in the risk of a range of HAI, a specific threshold level of adherence remains uncertain. In the absence of this standard, the aim across healthcare is to achieve 100% adherence.

The true standard for effective hand hygiene is not just quantitative performance of the frequency of opportunities met, but also the degree of focus attended to each individual opportunity. The WHO has identified 5 separate "moments" for hand hygiene associated with each patient contact (Fig. 1.3). Meticulous adherence to recommended usage for the full range of hand hygiene products (including soap and water as well as alcohol-based hand rubs) is crucial.

The use of **personal protective equipment** extends the concept of physical barriers to transmission. The donning of disposable gowns and gloves has been associated with a reduction in the spread of MDROs, especially in the setting of an outbreak. As a result, PPE is recommended as a central element of most recommendations and standards for the control of MDROs.

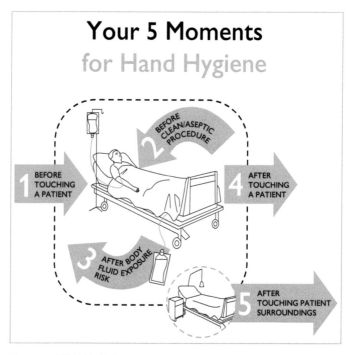

Figure 1.3 World Health Organization 5 moments for hand hygiene

By preventing the transmission of pathogens on the clothes and hands of healthcare personnel, PPE offers an attractive and sensible supplement to hand hygiene. However, some concerns have been raised about whether patients placed in isolation precautions may be at greater risk for patient safety events and declining mental status.

Environmental controls can be applied to further extend the barriers that protect patients from the transmission of HAI. Some of these controls are simplistic, including the placement of patients with specific infectious syndromes into bed spaces that are appropriate for the prevention of spread. Examples include the use of negative-pressure rooms for patients with tuberculosis and single-patient rooms for individuals with MDRO(s).

More refined approaches to environmental control emerge from the awareness that inanimate surfaces and equipment in hospitals can themselves serve as a fomite source for the transmission of MDROs and other pathogens. Patients assigned to hospital rooms previously occupied by individuals colonized or infected with a specific MDRO are themselves at increased risk for acquisition of the same pathogen, even after adjusting for other confounding variables. Timely and meticulous room cleaning, particularly when room occupancy is being changed (terminal clean) may reduce the risk of infection in some circumstances.

Mitigating the Risk of Serious Infection

It has long been established that despite the deployment of basic transmission control measures, hospitalized patients may nevertheless become colonized with pathogens that pose a threat for subsequent infection, especially in the setting of compromise of host defenses. There is increasing evidence that the risk of deep infection with these potentially lethal pathogens can be reduced through a number of basic bedside interventions.

Empiric evidence has revealed a series of **best practices for the management of invasive devices** that are associated with a risk of device-related infection and complication. Perhaps the best evidence has emerged from the experience with central vascular access devices. In this case, a bundle of interventions has been developed, studied, and deployed. For the most part, these practices are designed to reduce the risk of catheter colonization and the migration of pathogens into the endovascular system. Although the evidence in support of some individual elements of this bundle has been questioned, the impact of the bundle when deployed together in association with concurrent efforts to improve the culture of safety and enhance communication can have dramatic effects. Similar bundles have now been proposed for the prevention of ventilator-associated pneumonia and catheter-associated urinary tract infection.

Decolonization and antimicrobial strategies are proposed as a more direct means of limiting the impact of virulent or resistant colonizing strains of hospital-associated bacteria. Fundamentally, the aim with this approach is to unburden the host of the more threatening microbes and to eventually reestablish the benign colonization barrier that typically protects us. Historical efforts have ranged from the administration of systemic antibiotics to selective gut decontamination. More recently, considerable strides have been made in the application of more targeted measures. A later chapter discusses the impact of mupirocin to reduce the risk of infection with *S. aureus*, and especially those strains that are resistant to methicillin. A further and more recent extension of this approach is the application of chlorhexidine baths to patients in the ICU as a means to reduce the risk of central line-associated bloodstream infection (CLABSI).

The role of chlorhexidine as a skin disinfectant has already been established in other settings. As was noted chlorhexidine skin preparation is an important element of the bundle of interventions to prevent CLABSI. In addition, chlorhexidine-based preparations have been found to be superior to povidone-iodine solutions as skin preparation before most surgeries. Indeed, much of surgical practice is centered on techniques to mitigate the risk of infection to the host. Examples include perioperative glycemic control and periprocedural antibiotic prophylaxis.

Suggested Reading

Allegranzi B, Pittet D. Role of hand hygiene in healthcare-associated infection prevention. J Hosp Infect 2009;73(4):305–315.

Carboneau C, Benge E, Jaco MT, Robinson M. A lean Six Sigma team increases hand hygiene compliance and reduces hospital-acquired MRSA infections by 51%. J Healthc Qual 2010;32(4):61–70.

Datta R, Platt R, Yokoe DS, Huang SS. Environmental cleaning intervention and risk of acquiring multidrug-resistant organisms from prior room occupants. Arch Intern Med 2011;171:491–494.

Dellit TH, Owens RC, McGowan JE, Gerding DN, Weinstein RA, Burke JP, et al. Infectious Diseases Society of America and the Society for Healthcare Epidemiology of America guidelines for developing an institutional program to enhance antimicrobial stewardship. Clin Infect Dis 2007;44:159–177.

Hebert C, Robicsek A. Decolonization therapy in infection control. Curr Opin Infect Dis 2010;23:340–345.

Jernigan JA, Titus MG, Gröschel DH, Getchell-White S, Farr BM. Effectiveness of contact isolation during a hospital outbreak of methicillin-resistant Staphylococcus aureus. Am J Epidemiol 1996;143(5):496–504.

Parker J, ed. Risk assessment for infection prevention and control. Oakbrook Terrace, IL: Joint Commission Resources, 2010.

Pronovost P, Needham D, Berenholtz S, Sinopoli D, Chu H, Cosgrove S, et al. An intervention to decrease catheter-related bloodstream infections in the ICU. NEJM 2006;355:2725–2732.

Pittet D, Hugonnet S, Harbarth S, Mourouga P, Sauvan V, Touveneau S, et al. Effectiveness of a hospital-wide programme to improve compliance with hand hygiene. Infection Control Programme. Lancet 2000;356:1307–1312.

Stelfox HT, Bates DW, Redelmeier DA. Safety of patients isolated for infection control. JAMA 2003;290:1899–905.

Chapter 2a

Ventilator-Associated Pneumonia

Curtis J. Coley II and Melissa A. Miller

Initial Case Presentation

M.L. is a 77 year-old male with a history of rheumatoid arthritis on chronic prednisone, previous myocardial infarction, and congestive heart failure, who presents to the emergency department with respiratory distress and chest pressure. He appears cyanotic and is lethargic. He is afebrile, with a blood pressure of 220/115 and a respiratory rate of 35. His room air oxygen saturation is 60%. He is urgently intubated and placed on mechanical ventilation. Initial laboratory values include a normal troponin level and white blood cell count, with an elevated B-type natriuretic peptide of 1,800 pg/ml. Portable chest radiography shows bilateral vascular congestion consistent with pulmonary edema. He is admitted to the Coronary Care Unit for further management. Because of the patient's inability to breathe in coordination with the ventilator, continuous infusion of a paralytic agent is required to maintain adequate oxygenation. Over the next several days, with diuresis and blood pressure control, the patient improves significantly. The paralytic is discontinued on hospital day 3. At this time, the attending physician notices that the head of the patient's bed is not elevated. Nursing notes reveal that the patient has been lying flat for the previous 24 hours after a procedure was performed.

On hospital day 4, M.L. becomes febrile to 40°C. His blood pressure is 80/40. He has an increased oxygen requirement, and copious amounts of thick yellow sputum have been suctioned from the endotracheal tube over the past several hours. A STAT portable chest radiograph demonstrates resolving vascular congestion, with a new focal left lower lobe opacity (Figure 2.1). Labs are notable for an elevated white blood cell count of 15,000/mm³.

Differential Diagnosis

The differential diagnosis for new pulmonary infiltrates and fever in a patient requiring mechanical ventilation is broad and includes pneumonia, aspiration pneumonitis, atelectasis, pulmonary embolism, malignancy, and acute respiratory distress syndrome (ARDS). Because the approach to management of each of these entities varies, it is important for the clinician to make the correct diagnosis in order to initiate appropriate therapy. The elevated white blood

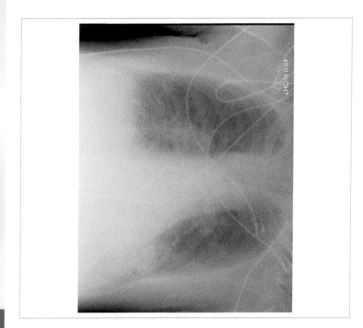

Figure 2.1 Chest radiograph of an intubated patient with left lower lobe infiltrate.

cell count, increase in sputum production, and increased oxygen requirement in this case suggest a diagnosis of pneumonia, specifically, ventilator-associated pneumonia (VAP).

There are three different classifications of nosocomial pneumonia. Hospital-acquired pneumonia (HAP) is defined as pneumonia identified 48 hours or more after admission to the hospital that was not incubating at the time of admission. Ventilator-associated pneumonia is defined as pneumonia in a patient who is or who has been endotracheally intubated within the last 48 hours. Healthcare-associated pneumonia (HCAP) can occur in any patient who was hospitalized in an acute care hospital for 2 or more days within 90 days of the infection; resided in a nursing home or long-term care facility; received recent intravenous anti-biotic therapy, chemotherapy, or wound care within the past 30 days of infection; or received hemodialysis in a clinic or hospital setting. The microbiology of HCAP has been shown to be more similar to HAP and VAP compared with that of community-acquired pneumonia. The vast majority of causative organisms for HAP and VAP are bacterial, most commonly gram-positive cocci and/or gram-negative rods including *Staphylococcus aureus* and methicillin resistant *S. aureus* [MRSA], *Streptococcus* spp., *Escherichia coli*, *Klebsiella pneumonia*, *Enterobacter* spp., *Pseudomonas aeruginosa*, and *Acinetobacter* spp. *S. aureus*, *P. aeruginosa*, *K. pneumo*, and *E. coli* account for more than half of cases.

Cases of HAP have been reported to occur at a rate between 5 and 10 cases per 1,000 hospital admissions, with the incidence increasing by as much as 6- to 20-fold in mechanically ventilated patients. Other risk factors for VAP include

advanced age, underlying illness, aspiration, prolonged intubation or reintuba-
tion, a diagnosis of ARDS, and the continuous use of paralytic agents. Our patient had several of these risk factors. The crude mortality rate of nosocomial
pneumonia has been reported to be between 20% and 50%. Increased mortality
has been associated with those cases complicated by bacteremia, especially
with *Pseudomonas* and *Acinetobacter* species, medical rather than surgical illness, and treatment with ineffective antibiotic therapy. Overall, a diagnosis of
VAP is associated with longer intensive care unit and hospital length of stay,
leading to higher crude hospital costs compared with uninfected patients, ranging from $10,000 to more than $40,000 per episode. After adjusting for illness
severity, the attributable cost of VAP is estimated to average nearly $10,000 to
$14,000 per case. Additionally, uncontrolled VAP can lead to morbid condi-
tions such as empyema and lung abscess, longer intubation times, and additional
procedures including tracheostomy placement.

To diagnose nosocomial pneumonia, there must be a new or worsening infiltrate on chest imaging, as well as clinical characteristics such as fever, purulent
sputum, leukocytosis, and a decline in oxygenation. Our patient manifested all
of these characteristics. Microbiological criteria for the diagnosis of HAP/VAP
require the clinical criteria with the addition of specimen sampling of the lower
respiratory tract with positive culture. In contrast, there has been no evidence
to date showing a benefit in lower respiratory sampling in the absence of any
clinical indicator of pneumonia, and this practice may lead to unnecessary treatment, contribute to drug-resistant epidemiology, and expose patients to antibiotic side effects in the absence of clinical benefit.

There are various methods used to sample the microorganisms of the lower
airway. These are typically divided into two categories: bronchoscopic and nonbronchoscopic approaches. Bronchoscopic sampling includes bronchoalveolar lavage (BAL) and protected brush sampling. Nonbronchoscopic sampling
methods include tracheobronchial aspiration and mini-BAL. Table 2.1 outlines
the various sampling methods in further detail. The advantages of bronchoscopic methods include visually-directed sampling, higher specificity in culture
results, and thus the potential of allowing for more rapid narrowing of antibiotic
therapy.

Conversely, nonbronchoscopic methods do not require a high level of clinical expertise and thus can be obtained more quickly at a lower cost. Also, they
allow for multiple samples over time if needed. Though one study showed a
slight mortality benefit in patients undergoing bronchoscopic sampling, this has
not been reproduced in other studies. Bronchoscopic sampling should be performed if possible; however, in its absence nonbronchoscopic sampling should
be performed in an effort to identify the microbiologic pathogen responsible
for the pneumonia and to tailor antibiotic therapy to accurate susceptibility
information.

Quantitative culture thresholds have been recommended to aid in the diagnosis of VAP (see Table 2.1). Though these thresholds are intended to decrease
the likelihood of false-negative results, their use has not been shown to improve
any clinical outcome compared with semiquantitative cultures (i.e., heavy, moderate, light, or no bacterial growth), where heavy to moderate growth is considered positive.

Table 2.1 Description of Bronchoscopic and Nonbronchoscopic Sampling Methods, and their Respective Thresholds for a Positive Quantitative Culture

Sampling Method	Procedure Description	Threshold for a Positive Quantitative Culture in Colony Forming Units/ milliliter (CFU/ml)
Protected Specimen Brush (PSB)	A sheathed brush is pushed through a bronchoscope until the sheath is adjacent to the desired airway. A specimen is collected by brushing the airway wall.	$>10^3$
Bronchoalveolar Lavage (BAL)	Infusion and aspiration of sterile saline are done through a bronchoscope that is wedged into a bronchial segment.	$>10^4$
Tracheobronchial Aspiration	A catheter is advanced through the endotracheal tube until resistance is met, then suction is applied to the catheter.	$>10^5$
Mini-BAL	A catheter is advanced through the endotracheal tube until resistance is met. Sterile saline is infused through the catheter and then aspirated.	$>10^5$

Case Presentation (continued)

In response to the patient's declining clinical condition and infiltrates observed on chest radiography, the intensivist orders administration of intravenous fluids and vasopressors. Two sets of blood cultures and a mini-BAL specimen are also collected. The physician also orders piperacillin/tazobactam and vancomycin for the empiric treatment of VAP. Within 12 hours of providing the laboratory with samples, both the blood cultures and mini-BAL demonstrate gram-negative bacilli on gram staining. At this time, the patient remains febrile and is now requiring 1.00 FiO2 in order to maintain his oxygen saturation greater than 90%.

Management and Discussion

As stated, the most common microorganisms responsible for HAP and VAP are gram-positive cocci (e.g., *Staphylococcus aureus*, including MRSA, and *Streptococcus* spp.), and gram-negative bacilli (e.g., *Escherichia coli*, *Klebsiella pneumoniae*, *Enterobacter* spp., *Pseudomonas aeruginosa*, *Acinetobacter* spp.).

Generally, infections with multidrug-resistant organisms (i.e., Pseudomonas, Acinetobacter), bacteremia with the causative organism, and multilobar or cavitating disease cause more complications and worse clinical outcomes.

In our case, the physician's rapid correction of hypotension, microbiological sampling, and initiation of broad-spectrum antibiotics is appropriate. The vast majority of causative organisms would be covered by these particular agents. Microbes that potentially would not be covered by this empiric regimen are multidrug-resistant (MDR) gram negatives. The definition of multi-drug resistance varies depending on the source; however, CDC defines these organisms as resistant to at least one class of antimicrobial agent to which the organism is usually susceptible. Patient risk factors for infection with MDR organisms include: receipt of antibiotics within the preceding 90 days, current hospitalization of 5 days or more, high frequency of antibiotic resistance in the community or specific hospital, and patient immunosuppression. VAP caused by an MDR pathogen is of some concern in this case because the patient receives chronic prednisone for rheumatoid arthritis.

The presence and type of MDR pathogen are variable, and it is important for clinicians to be familiar with susceptibility patterns in their respective facilities. In institutions in which there is a high frequency of resistant gram-negative organisms, clinicians should strongly consider empiric coverage with agents from two different antibiotic classes commonly effective against these pathogens. Recommendations for treatment of HAP, VAP, and HCAP are summarized in Figure 2.2.

Given our patient's chronic immunosuppression, a reasonable addition to the regimen in this case would have been an aminoglycoside or an anti-pseudomonal fluoroquinolone. Depending on the epidemiology of the institution, use of a carbapenem-based therapeutic regimen may have been indicated for resistant gram-negative organisms, especially in the setting of a high institutional prevalence of MDR organisms, such as extended spectrum β-lactamase-producing Enterobacteriaceae, β-lactam resistant *Pseudomonas* spp., or *Acinetobacter* spp.

Coverage for resistant gram-positive organisms, specifically MRSA, should be considered in patients with risk factors for MRSA, such as previous use of antibiotics, HIV infection, hemodialysis, and residence in a long-term care facility. Patients who are known to be colonized with MRSA should also be empirically covered for this organism. Coverage also should be strongly considered in communities with a high prevalence of community-acquired MRSA infections and in patients who are critically ill. Vancomycin remains first-line therapy for MRSA in most institutions; however, linezolid has been shown in some trials to have a higher rate of treatment success for VAP and may be considered for empiric therapy. Additionally, MRSA strains with rising vancomycin MICs (>1) are more likely to be treated inadequately with vancomycin, even with higher doses. In patients with known colonization with these strains or in institutions where these strains are prevalent, linezolid should be more strongly considered. These last two points further illustrate the need for clinicians to be aware of resistance patterns in their local areas.

Duration of antibiotics in the setting of VAP depend on the organism isolated and the patient's clinical response. If there is significant improvement in

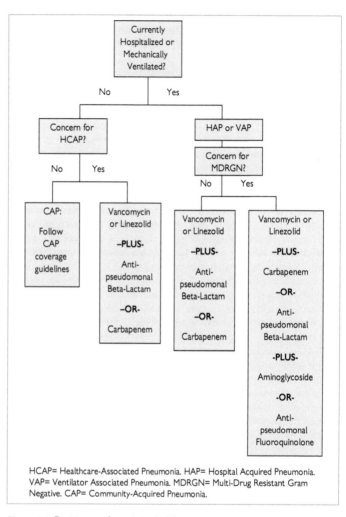

HCAP= Healthcare-Associated Pneumonia. HAP= Hospital Acquired Pneumonia. VAP= Ventilator Associated Pneumonia. MDRGN= Multi-Drug Resistant Gram Negative. CAP= Community-Acquired Pneumonia.

Figure 2.2 Decision tree for antimicrobial therapy.

the first 72 hours of antibiotic administration, an organism is obtained, and the empiric regimen was adequate, 7 to 8 total days of antibiotic therapy is sufficient. However, extended therapy (15–21 days) may be indicated for pseudomonal infection, complicated MRSA infection, and in the absence of clinical improvement in the first 72 hours.

Because VAP is associated with a significant degree of morbidity and mortality, a major goal of clinical care should be prevention. Lorente et al. presented an exhaustive list of prevention recommendations along with supporting evidence. In summary, patient placement in a semirecumbent position (elevation of the head of the bed to greater than 30 degrees), chlorhexidine oral rinse in combination with thorough mechanical cleaning of the oral cavity, avoidance of deep sedation and/or paralysis when possible, and daily assessment for extubation readiness are all steps that can decrease the incidence of VAP.

Case Conclusion

Over the next 24 hours, M.L.'s condition continues to worsen. He requires increasing doses of vasopressors to maintain mean arterial pressures above 65 mmHg. On hospital day 6, cultures confirm MDR-*Acinetobacter*, resistant to piperacillin/tazobactam, and susceptible only to tobramycin and imipenem. With this new information, the physician changes to an appropriate antibiotic regimen and continues aggressive management. On hospital day 7, the patient becomes bradycardic, with an oxygen saturation of 40% despite maximal support. He then experiences a PEA arrest. Advanced cardiac life support measures are initiated and maintained for 45 minutes without return of spontaneous circulation. The patient is declared deceased.

Suggested Reading

ATS/IDSA. Guidelines for management of adults with hospital-acquired, ventilator-associated, and healthcare-associated pneumonia. Am J Respir Crit Care Med 2005;171:388–416.

Chastre J, Fagon JY. Ventilator-associated pneumonia. Am J Respir Crit Care Med 2002;165:867–903.

Lorente L, Blot S, Rello J. Evidence on measures for the prevention of ventilator-associated pneumonia. Eur Respir J 2007;30:1193–1207.

Rello J, Ollendorf DA, Oster G, Vera-Llonch M, Bellm L, Redman R, et al. Epidemiology and outcomes of ventilator-associated pneumonia in a large US database. Chest 2002;122:2115–2121.

Tablan OC, Anderson LJ, Besser R, Bridges C, Hajjeh R. Guidelines for preventing health-care–associated pneumonia, 2003: recommendations of CDC and the Healthcare Infection Control Practices Advisory Committee. MMWR Recomm Rep 2004;53:1–36.

Chapter 2b

Aspiration Pneumonia

Pranavi Sreeramoju

Initial Case Presentation

A 45-year old male patient is admitted to the telemetry unit for mental confusion, agitation, fluctuating levels of consciousness, and increased heart and respiratory rates. He was previously healthy except for a history of alcohol abuse. The admitting physician diagnoses him with severe acute alcohol withdrawal syndrome. He is treated with intravenous lorazepam infusion titrated to his level of consciousness, hydration, and multiple B vitamins including 100mg of thiamine daily. On the fourth day of his hospital stay, the benzodiazepine medication is transitioned to oral chlordiazepoxide as he becomes more alert. He is transferred to the medicine ward where he continues to improve.

Just before his planned discharge on hospital day 6, the nurse notes him to be tachycardic and tachypneic. A check of his temperature reveals a fever of 39.4°C. His physical examination is impressive for new crackles heard in both the lung bases, more prominently on the right side. In contrast, his abdominal exam remains unremarkable. He does not have calf swelling or tenderness, or pitting pedal edema. When contacted, the physician orders blood work and a chest radiograph. When the results are returned several hours later, the patient's peripheral white blood cell count has increased from 10 to 15 cells per mm³. The chest radiograph is similar to the image shown in Figure 2.3. The patient continues to appear uncomfortable with increasingly labored breathing.

Differential Diagnosis and Initial Management

Aspiration is a major cause of pneumonia in the healthcare setting. Aspiration pneumonia refers to the clinical syndrome and radiological abnormality that develop after the unexpected entry of oropharyngeal or gastric contents and accompanying bacterial flora into the lower airways. Pneumonia occurs in approximately 250,000 hospitalized patients annually in the United States, accounting for 15% of all healthcare-associated infections.[1] Aspiration contributes to a significant majority of these infections, although the exact proportion is unknown.[2] Incidentally, aspiration pneumonia also accounts for 7 to 24% of community-acquired pneumonia cases and up to 30% of pneumonia occurring in continuing care facilities.[3] Aspiration pneumonia among hospital inpatients is associated with prolonged length of hospital stay by 7 to 9 days on average, excess healthcare costs of more than $40,000 per patient, and up to 30% increased risk of death.[2]

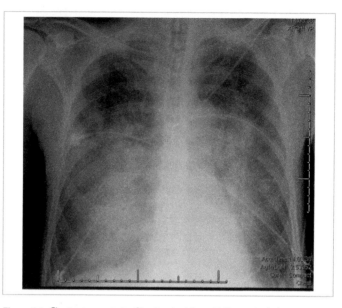

Figure 2.3 Chest anteroposterior film showing bilateral infiltrates in the lung parenchyma, more pronounced in the right lung.

(Image courtesy of Paul E. Marik, MD, Eastern Virginia Medical School, Norfolk, VA.)

In general, pneumonia in the healthcare setting can be further categorized as hospital-acquired pneumonia (HAP), ventilator-associated pneumonia (discussed separately in this book), and healthcare-associated pneumonia (HCAP). Strictly speaking, HAP has been defined as lower respiratory tract infection that occurs 48 hours or more after hospital admission in the absence of signs or symptoms of previously incubating infection. The definition of HCAP is described as lower respiratory tract infection occurring in patients with close contact with the healthcare system, recognized by the presence of at least one of the following risk factors: history of recent hospitalization or residence in a nursing home or extended care facility within 90 days of symptom onset, receipt of dialysis, home infusion therapy or wound care within 30 days of symptom onset, or living with someone with a multi-drug resistant pathogen. The pathophysiological prerequisites for development of aspiration pneumonia are compromise in host defenses that protect the airway such as cough and the gag reflex, accompanied by entry of a sufficient bacterial inoculum or obstruction by particulate matter with subsequent development of clinical signs of infection.

Aspiration pneumonia must be distinguished from two other common syndromes that occur following aspiration of gastric contents: aspiration pneumonitis and diffuse aspiration bronchiolitis.[4] Aspiration pneumonitis is defined as acute lung injury following the aspiration of regurgitated gastric contents. Diffuse aspiration bronchiolitis, on the other hand, occurs because of recurrent

occheral aspiration, usually in the elderly and occasionally in the middle-aged population. It should be suspected in older patients with recurrent episodes of
bronchorrhea, bronchospasm, and dyspnea. These two conditions are noninfectious and antimicrobial treatment is not indicated.

Pathogens commonly associated with aspiration pneumonia among hospitalized patients are generally those that colonize the oropharynx (Table 2.2). Many
of these infections are polymicrobial, representing the heterogeneous nature

Table 2.2 Suspected Pathogens causing Aspiration Pneumonia and Choices for Empiric Antimicrobial Therapy

Patients without Risk Factors for MDR Pathogens
Suspected Pathogens:

- *Streptococcus pneumoniae*
- *Hemophilus influenzae*
- Methicillin-susceptible *Staphylococcus aureus*
- Antimicrobial susceptible enteric gram negative bacilli:
- *Escherichia coli*
- *Klebsiella pneumoniae*
- *Enterobacter* species
- *Proteus* species
- *Serratia marcescens*

Empiric Antimicrobial Therapy Options

• Ceftriaxone	or
• Ciprofloxacin	or
• Moxifloxacin	or
• Levofloxacin	or
• Ertapenem	or
• Ampicillin/ Sulbactam	

Patients with Risk Factors for MDR Pathogens
Suspected Pathogens:

- Methicillin-resistant *Staphylococcus aureus* (MRSA)
- Antimicrobial resistant enteric gram negative bacilli listed to the left
- *K.pneumoniae* or *E.coli* with extended-spectrum ß lactamase (ESBL)
- *Pseudomonas aeruginosa*
- Carbapenem-resistant *Enterobacteriaceae*
- *Legionella pneumophila*

Empiric Antimicrobial therapy Options

• Antipseudomonal cephalosporin (Cefepime, Ceftazidime)	or
• Antipseudomonal carbapenem (Imipenem, Meropenem)	or
• β-lactam/β-lactamase inhibitor (Piperacillin/ Tazobactam)	

AND (for double coverage for gram-negative bacteria)

• Fluoroquinolone (Ciprofloxacin, Levofloxacin, Moxifloxacin)	or
• Aminoglycoside (Amikacin, Gentamicin, Tobramycin)	or

AND (for MRSA coverage)

• Linezolid	or
• Vancomycin	

Antimicrobials must be de-escalated to the narrowest possible spectrum immediately upon
availability of culture and susceptibility results.

of the flora typically found at this site. Surprisingly, the anaerobic bacteria typically recognized as an important part of the oral flora have a less important role in the development of aspiration pneumonia in hospitalized patients. This is likely attributable to the common overgrowth and oropharyngeal colonization of hospitalized patients with aerobic bacteria. When anaerobic pathogens are recovered from patients with aspiration pneumonia, common pathogens include *Peptostreptococcus*, *Fusobacterium nucleatum*, *Prevotella*, and *Bacteroides* species.

Risk factors for developing aspiration pneumonia include impaired consciousness, dysphagia from neurological deficits, gastroesophageal reflux disease, and mechanical injury to the upper respiratory tract (generally caused by intubation). The diagnosis of aspiration pneumonia is largely based on the presence of clinical symptoms and signs of pneumonia with supporting evidence from lower respiratory tract specimen cultures and chest radiography. However, the clinical presentation of even severe aspiration pneumonia may be highly variable, depending on host characteristics and the causative pathogen. If anaerobic bacteria are the cause of aspiration pneumonia, the clinical presentation is often notable for indolent symptoms, sometimes accompanied by sputum with putrid odor. The anatomic location of radiologic infiltrates is characteristically in the dependent pulmonary segments. Aspiration is more common in the right lung because the right main bronchus is straighter and shorter than the left main bronchus, favoring the distribution of aspirated material to this site. When aspiration occurs in the recumbent position, the infection may occur more typically in the superior segments of the lower lobes and the posterior segments of the upper lobes.

When aspiration pneumonia is suspected, lower respiratory tract samples (a good quality sputum specimen, endotracheal aspirate, or bronchoalveolar lavage, depending on the clinical situation) should ideally be obtained for microbiologic cultures before initiation of antimicrobial therapy. Empiric antimicrobial therapy may be deferred if the clinical suspicion for aspiration pneumonia is low or the preliminary microscopy of the lower respiratory specimen is unremarkable. The choice between narrow versus broad-spectrum empiric antimicrobial therapy is based on absence or presence of risk factors for multi-drug resistant (MDR) pathogens, and may be influenced by the severity of the patient's presentation (Table 2.2). Risk factors for MDR pathogens causing aspiration pneumonia in the healthcare setting include the previously noted risks for HCAP, receipt of antimicrobial therapy in the previous 3 months, delayed onset of symptoms relative to the day of admission ($\geq$5 days), high frequency of antimicrobial resistance based on antimicrobial susceptibility data from the hospital unit, and presence of immunosuppressive conditions. When such risk factors are present, published guidelines suggest the use of broad-spectrum combination therapies including double coverage for gram-negative bacteria and agents with activity against MRSA. However, empiric therapy should be tailored to cover the most likely causative pathogen(s), including microbes that have been identified as colonizing the patient's oropharynx. This approach should limit excessive use of empiric antibiotics. It is appropriate to add clindamycin or metronidazole if the other antimicrobials in the planned regimen do not have antianaerobic activity and anaerobic pathogens are suspected. If infection with

Legionella pneumophila is suspected (typically in the case of severe multilobar pneumonia of sudden onset), a macrolide or a fluoroquinolone also should be included. As is true for all patients with evidence of infection, the patient must be placed in appropriate isolation precautions based on pathogen(s) identified in concordance with the hospital policy. Evaluation for presence of complications must be done and dental consultation obtained if clinically indicated in order to reduce the risk of future recurrent infection.

Case Presentation (continued)

Based on the high clinical suspicion for aspiration pneumonia and low likelihood of MDR pathogens, sputum specimen for culture was obtained and empiric treatment was initiated with moxifloxacin to cover common gram-positive and gram-negative bacteria. Three days later, the patient's sputum culture grew *Klebsiella pneumoniae* that was susceptible to most antibiotics tested, including moxifloxacin. His blood cultures demonstrated no growth even after 5 days of incubation in the laboratory.

Management and Discussion

Further management of a patient with aspiration pneumonia such as the one described here depends on close clinical follow-up and the results of continued laboratory evaluation. A straightforward algorithm can be helpful to guide decisions (Fig. 2.4) Antimicrobial therapy can be deescalated to a narrow-spectrum alternative once culture and susceptibility results are available to exclude the

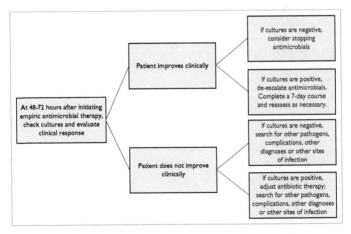

Figure 2.4 Algorithm to guide clinical decision-making at 48 to 72 hours after suspecting aspiration pneumonia.

(American Thoracic Society/ Infectious Diseases Society of America guidelines 2005.)

involvement of MDR pathogens. The typical duration of antimicrobial therapy for aspiration pneumonia is 7 to 8 days for most patients unless complications occur. There is a growing body of evidence to support even shorter duration (3–5 days) of antimicrobial therapies for mild to moderately severe pneumonia regardless of etiology.[6,7]

Potential complications of aspiration pneumonia include lung abscess, necrotizing pneumonia, parapneumonic effusion, and empyema secondary to bronchopleural fistula. Although relatively uncommon, any sign of persistent or progressive symptoms in the face of appropriate antimicrobial therapy should prompt an evaluation for these phenomena.

Preventive strategies for aspiration pneumonia among hospitalized patients include: maintenance of the head of the bed at greater than 30 degrees from horizontal to reduce the likelihood of passive aspiration, frequent and aggressive oral care including chlorhexidine mouth rinse for high-risk patients, the avoidance of unnecessary antimicrobial and sedative administration, and frequent suctioning of oropharyngeal secretions in patients with impaired swallowing.[5]

Case Conclusion

The patient improved with treatment with Moxifloxacin. He was discharged home on hospital day nine with instructions to complete a total 7-day course of moxifloxacin, taper of chlordiazepoxide over 3 additional days, and referral to alcohol rehabilitation services.

References

Klevens RM, Edwards JR, Richards CL Jr., et al. Estimating health care-associated infections and deaths in U.S. hospitals, 2002. Public Health Rep 2007;122:160–166.

ATS/IDSA. Guidelines for the management of adults with hospital-acquired, ventilator-associated, and healthcare-associated pneumonia. Am J Respir Crit Care Med 2005;171:388–416.

Reza Shariatzadeh M, Huang JQ, Marrie TJ. Differences in the features of aspiration pneumonia according to site of acquisition: community or continuing care facility. J Am Geriatr Soc 2006;54:296–302.

Marik PE. Pulmonary aspiration syndromes. Curr Opin Pulm Med 2011;17:148–154.

Tablan OC, Anderson LJ, Besser R, Bridges C, Hajjeh R. Guidelines for preventing health-care--associated pneumonia, 2003: recommendations of CDC and the Healthcare Infection Control Practices Advisory Committee. MMWR Recomm Rep 2004;53:1–36.

Li JZ, Winston LG, Moore DH, Bent S. Efficacy of short-course antibiotic regimens for community-acquired pneumonia: a meta-analysis. Am J Med. 2007;120(9):783–790.

Pugh RJ, Cooke RP, Dempsey G. Short course antibiotic therapy for Gram-negative hospital-acquired pneumonia in the critically ill. J Hosp Infect. 2010;74(4):337–343.

Chapter 2c

Healthcare-Associated Legionellosis

Jennifer C. Esbenshade and Thomas R. Talbot

Initial Case Presentation

The patient is a 52 year-old man who, as a result of a kerosene tank explosion, sustained full-thickness thermal burns on his abdomen and lower extremities (an estimated 40% of his body surface area). In the emergency department, his O_2 saturation was 97%, pulse 120 beats per minute, and blood pressure 80/20 mm Hg. Physical examination revealed a well-nourished man with full-thickness thermal burns over the legs and abdomen. There was no respiratory distress, hoarseness, or coughing. The remainder of the physical exam was normal.

In the emergency room, the patient was given aggressive fluid resuscitation and topical burn care. He was transferred to a regional burn center where treatment continued in accordance with current practice standards. The wounds underwent whirlpool debridement and hydrotherapy beginning on the seventh day of hospitalization.

Eleven days after admission, the patient began having a mild, intermittent productive cough and spiked a fever to 40°C. He also developed headache in a band distribution across the forehead, myalgias, and nausea. His respiratory rate increased to 22 breaths per minute. On physical examination, the patient was tachypneic but in no apparent distress. Breath sounds were decreased at the right base, and there were fine crackles with deep inspiration. His burns did not appear to demonstrate specific evidence of bacterial superinfection. The remainder of the physical exam was unchanged.

Differential Diagnosis and Initial Management

After several days in the intensive care unit, the patient has developed clinical signs and symptoms of pneumonia. Because symptoms began more than 48 hours after admission, the pneumonia may be considered to be hospital-acquired. When associated with infection within the first 5 days of hospital admission, causative bacterial pathogens are more likely to be antibiotic-susceptible, whereas a longer hospital stay before the onset of symptoms is generally associated with colonization and infection with multidrug-resistant gram-negative and gram-positive organisms (MDROs). Of course, if specific MDROs are common in a particular hospital unit, this should be taken into account and initial antibiotic coverage adjusted accordingly. A Gram stain of sputum may provide important information regarding the most likely microbiologic cause, and growth in culture of 10^5 bacteria per ml of sputum should be considered especially significant. In addition to sputum cultures, a blood culture may be considered as part of the evaluation of hospital-acquired pneumonia (HAP), although the yield is generally low for most organisms, with the exception of *Staphylococcus aureus* and *Staphylococcus pneumoniae*. A more complete discussion of the pathogens most commonly associated with HAP is included in the case and discussion of aspiration pneumonia.

In evaluating a patient with HAP, respiratory viruses transmitted from the hands or respiratory secretions of visitors or healthcare professionals also should be considered. In contrast, hospital-acquired pneumonia is rarely caused by fungal organisms in the immunocompetent host.

The differential diagnosis in this case should also include *Legionella* species. Although typically associated with severe community-acquired infection (particularly in the setting of clusters and outbreaks), this potentially lethal organism has the potential to contaminate hospital water supplies and has been reported as an important cause of outbreaks of infection in hospitals and other healthcare facilities. Participation in hydrotherapy could have exposed the patient to the pathogen if harbored within the hospital water system. To evaluate for legionellosis, a urinary antigen immunoassay can qualitatively detect the involvement of *Legionella* serogroup 1, which causes the majority of human infections. The sensitivity and specificity of this test for detecting serogroup 1 exceed 95%. Legionellosis is also associated with hyponatremia, elevated liver transaminases, elevated ferritin, and microscopic hematuria and proteinuria. To grow the organism, sputum must be cultured on buffered charcoal yeast extract agar in addition to routine culture media. Alerting the clinical microbiology laboratory of the suspicion for legionellosis is important.

Case Presentation (continued)

Laboratory evaluation ordered in the setting of the patient's fever and worsening respiratory status demonstrated a peripheral white blood cell count of 14,000/mm^3 with a differential count of 85% neutrophils, 10% lymphocytes, and 5% monocytes. The basic metabolic panel revealed sodium of 125 meq/L and phosphate of 0.5 mmol/L. Serum glutamic oxaloacetic transaminase was 110 U/L, serum glutamic pyruvic transaminase was 133 U/L; but the hepatic panel was otherwise normal. Serum ferritin was 700 ng/ml. A urinalysis revealed microscopic hematuria and 2+ proteinuria. Chest radiography showed patchy bilateral infiltrates in the lower lobes and a small right pleural effusion. The physician in the burn unit ordered that a sputum sample be sent for culture. Gram stain showed many neutrophils but no organisms. While awaiting the results of further testing, the physician ordered that vancomycin and piperacillin/tazobactam be administered in standard parenteral doses. Over the next 3 days, fever persisted, and the patient became more tachypneic, ultimately requiring supplemental oxygen via face mask. A repeat chest radiograph showed increasing consolidation in the right lower lobe (Fig. 2.5). A urinary antigen test for *Legionella* ordered on hospital day nine was positive.

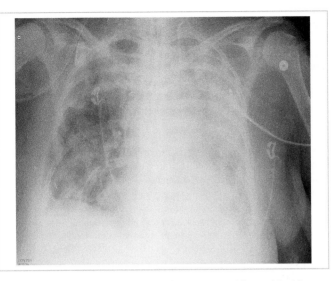

Figure 2.5 Chest radiograph demonstrating progressive consolidation of the right lower lobe.

Management and Discussion

The clinical presentation and laboratory findings are consistent with health-care-acquired legionellosis. *Legionella* species are gram-negative bacteria that inhabit freshwater sources and can contaminate potable water sources and stores. The bacterium was named after an outbreak of pneumonia-like illness affecting American Legionnaires attending a statewide convention in 1976 at the Belleview Stratford Hotel in Philadelphia (Fig. 2.6). The causative agent, *Legionella*, was discovered by James McDade in 1977. Although cooling towers have commonly been implicated in outbreaks of infection, as was the case in the 1976 Philadelphia outbreak, potable water remains the major environmental source for outbreaks in the community and institutions. In fact, the organism is considered a commensal in water systems of large buildings, and regular preventive maintenance is recommended to keep colonization at safe levels. The organism is not transmitted from person-to-person; therefore an outbreak is usually traced to a single point source.

Legionella pneumonia, if left untreated, is associated with a mortality of 14% to 50% depending on the virulence of the strain and host factors. Pontiac Fever, a milder infection caused by the same pathogen, is a self-limited illness marked by constitutional symptoms but no pneumonia.

Legionella is recognized as a rare but important cause of healthcare-acquired pneumonia, although the incidence is not well defined because accurate reporting of cases requires routine legionella-specific testing on site, and many institutions do not have the capability to sustain this approach. Species of *Legionella*

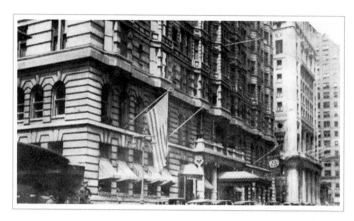

Figure 2.6 The Belleview Stratford Hotel (Philadelphia, PA) was the site of the first recognized outbreak of pneumonia ultimately attributed to legionellosis.

that are most commonly associated with HAP are *L. pneumophila*, *L. micdadei*, *L. sainhelense*, *L. bozmanii*, and *L. oakridgensis*. Potential sources in the health-care setting include aerosols generated for environmental control of temperature or humidity, respiratory therapy, and, as in this case, wound debridement. Exposure to the organism via intense aerosols generated for environmental control of temperature or humidity or medical procedures, such as those used in respiratory therapy and wound debridement, have been repeatedly implicated in outbreak investigations. Although the organism has also been cultured from hospital shower heads and sinks, the link between routine exposure to contaminated water from these sources and disease is less well established.

Colonization of the oropharynx and microaspiration into the pulmonary tree is thought to be a key step in the pathogenesis of most cases of healthcare-acquired legionellosis. Because of the likely underappreciated burden of healthcare-acquired legionellosis owing to limitations of laboratory testing and the nonspecific nature of some of the symptoms, a single case in a healthcare facility should be viewed as a possible sentinel event, indicating the potential for an occult source of exposure in the institution as well as additional undiscovered cases. If more than one case is identified, molecular subtyping can be used to compare strains and evaluate the possibility of a single environmental source of exposure.

To minimize *Legionella* colonization in the water supply of healthcare facilities, CDC environmental control guidelines state that cold water should be stored and distributed at temperatures below 20°C and hot water tank temperatures should be maintained above 60°C and circulated with a minimum return temperature of 51°C, or at the highest temperature specified in local regulations or building codes. In an outbreak, the most promising method of disinfection appears to be use of a copper-silver ionization system; however, other methods including chlorine dioxide and monochloramine are under investigation. An alternative method, "superheat and flush," involves raising the building water temperature to 70°C and flushing the entire system. Older hyperchlorination techniques are increasingly considered obsolete because of high cost, concerns about occupational safety, and concerns about reduced effectiveness in inhibiting long-term colonization.

Routine environmental monitoring for *Legionella* by culture followed by clinical surveillance among patients with HAP is controversial. Currently, the CDC recommends targeted surveillance among patients with HAP and does not recommend routine environmental cultures of hospital water systems unless an increased number of cases in the institution is detected.

Based on data from clinical trials, the newer macrolides, especially azithromycin, and fluoroquinolones have been shown to be most effective in treating legionellosis. Because the organism is not transmitted person-to-person, isolation precautions are not necessary for hospitalized patients.

Case Conclusion

After the *Legionella* urinary antigen test was reported as positive, the Infectious Diseases Consultant recommended that treatment be narrowed to azithromycin monotherapy. Within 2 days, the respiratory status of the patient improved. *Legionella pneumophila* ultimately grew from the sputum cultured on buffered charcoal yeast extract agar, confirming the diagnosis of legionellosis. The hospital's infection control team initiated an investigation to identify the potential source. Surveillance cultures were obtained from the hydrotherapy system, which was temporarily closed while the investigation was ongoing. When these specimens revealed the presence of a high growth of *Legionella*, the system was disinfected. No other cases were identified, even in the face of rigorous surveillance and testing of all hospitalized patients with new onset of respiratory complaints.

The patient was ultimately discharged after a month in the hospital. He is currently undergoing physical therapy and remains free of evidence of infection.

Suggested Reading

Centers for Disease Control and Prevention Healthcare Infection Control Practices Advisory Committee (HICPAC). Guidelines for environmental infection control in health-care facilities. MMWR 2003;52(RR10);1–42.

Niederman MS, Craven DE, et al. Guidelines for the management of adults with hospital-acquired, ventilator-associated, and healthcare-associated pneumonia. Am J Respir Crit Care Med 2005;171:388–416.

Sabria M and Yu VL. Hospital-acquired legionellosis: solutions for a preventable infection. Lancet Infect Dis 2002;2:368–373.

Stout JE et al. Role of environmental surveillance in determining the risk of hospital-acquired legionellosis: a national surveillance study with clinical correlations. Infect Control Hosp Epidemiol 2007;28(7):818–824.

Chapter 2d

Healthcare-Associated Viral Pneumonia

Jennifer C. Esbenshade and Thomas R. Talbot

Initial Case Presentation

An 8-month-old preterm baby boy with severe chronic lung disease and secondary pulmonary hypertension underwent tracheostomy in early January. He tolerated the procedure well and there were no evident complications. The patient was born at 28 weeks gestation, weighing 591 grams, and was immediately placed on a ventilator. During the first 6 months of his hospitalization, he completed recommended vaccinations against diphtheria, tetanus, pertussis, polio, pneumococcus, *Haemophilus influenzae* b and hepatitis B. A tunneled central venous catheter was inserted for long-term intravenous access.

On the seventh postoperative day, the bedside nurse noted a fever of 39.2°C. That morning, she also noted that his tracheal secretions had become thick and yellow and he required an increase in FiO2 through the ventilator. Her examination revealed a somnolent infant with tracheostomy connected to a ventilator. There was no erythema or drainage surrounding the tracheostomy site. There was no nasal discharge, and his conjunctivae were not injected. The infant's mucous membranes were moist and without lesions. Breath sounds were equal and symmetric, and there were diffuse crackles bilaterally. There was no heart murmur. Bowel sounds were distant, and the abdomen was distended. Brachial and pedal pulses were 1+ bilaterally and capillary refill was 5 seconds. The remainder of the physical exam was unchanged. The nurse contacted the attending physician to notify her of the change in the patient's status.

Differential Diagnosis and Initial Management

The onset of fever suggests an acute infectious process, and increased tracheal secretions and oxygen requirements localize illness to the lower respiratory tract. In addition to pneumonia, the differential diagnosis in this preterm infant with an indwelling venous catheter also includes catheter-related bloodstream infection and necrotizing entercolitis, both common entities in this vulnerable population. Although he recently had a tracheostomy procedure, there is no obvious sign of a surgical site infection. Based on clinical, laboratory, and radiographic findings, the case would appear to meet CDC surveillance-based definitions for ventilator-associated pneumonia. However, using such strict definitions is especially challenging in children with certain underlying comorbidities such as chronic lung disease related to prematurity and congenital heart disease that can confound clinical and radiographic findings.

In the ventilated patient, pneumonia may develop from organisms that are part of the patient's normal flora or after exposure to other pathogens via contaminated hands of healthcare personnel (HCP) or to contagious infections spread by respiratory droplets from infected staff, family members, or visitors. Bacterial pathogens that are commonly suspected to cause pneumonia in the intensive care unit setting include methicillin-susceptible and -resistant staphylococci, enteric gram negatives such as *Klebsiella pneumoniae*, *Escherichia coli*, and Enterobacter species, nontypeable *Haemophilus influenzae*, oral anaerobic pathogens, and endemic organisms such as *Pseudomonas aeruginosa* and *Acinetobacter baumannii*. Viral pathogens account for only about 20% of healthcare-associated viral pneumonias but should also be considered, especially during the winter months when annual community epidemics of respiratory syncytial virus (RSV) and influenza increase the likelihood that a visitor or HCP could shed virus either symptomatically or asymptomatically. Although influenza and RSV are the most commonly recognized respiratory viruses transmitted in the healthcare setting, nosocomial spread of other respiratory viruses including adenovirus, parainfluenza virus, human metapneumovirus, rhinovirus, and coronavirus have been reported. Seasonal variation in circulating viruses make certain pathogens more or less likely; for example influenza and RSV usually circulate from late fall to early spring, and adenovirus and parainfluenza viruses circulate year-round (Fig. 2.7).

To evaluate potential causes of deterioration in this patient, specimens should be sent for a complete blood count, a comprehensive metabolic panel, and routine bacterial cultures. A tracheal aspirate should be sent for Gram stain and bacterial, anaerobic, and viral cultures. Radiographs of both the chest and abdomen also should be obtained. Isolation of a viral pathogen is usually helpful in the hospitalized patient, and rapid antigen and multiplex nucleic acid assays are available to test for influenza and RSV. For influenza, PCR is most sensitive, but starting the diagnostic work-up with a rapid antigen test is reasonable because, although less sensitive (50%–86%), such assays are typically specific (96%–98%) when used during the winter respiratory virus season. Of note, the rapid antigen test has been reported to be less sensitive in young children (63%–74%) and older adults (19%–27%), and for certain strains of influenza such as 2009 H1N1 (40%–69%). If the causative organism is not readily determined by the above methods, bronchoscopy may be considered on an individual patient basis.

Case Presentation (continued)

The neonatologist, in conjunction with the Infectious Diseases Consultant, ordered a comprehensive workup to evaluate the respiratory deterioration. The peripheral white blood cell count was 36,800/mm^3 with a differential count of 70% neutrophils, 20% lymphocytes, and 10% monocytes. The basic metabolic panel was normal. The hepatic panel showed SGOT of 142 U/L but was otherwise normal. Spinal fluid and blood cultures were obtained, and empiric broad-spectrum antibacterial therapy was initiated.

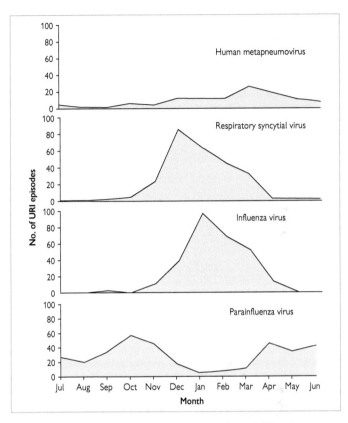

Figure 2.7 Epidemiologic pattern of upper respiratory infection (URI) respiratory viruses from 20 years of surveillance in the Vanderbilt Vaccine Clinic.

(JV Williams et al. The role of human metapneumovirus in upper respiratory tract infections in children: a 20-year experience. J Infect Dis 2006;193(3):387–395)

A chest radiograph demonstrated changes of severe chronic lung disease with upper lung zone and perihilar atelectasis, air trapping at the lung bases, enlarged cardiac silhouette, and a small left pleural effusion (Fig. 2.8). An abdominal radiograph did not demonstrate intraperitoneal free air, pneumatosis intestinalis, or portal venous gas suggestive of necrotizing enterocolitis. A rapid influenza test was sent and reported positive for influenza A. After referring to up to date CDC guidelines for antiviral therapy, which are based on patterns of antiviral resistance for circulating influenza strains, oseltamivir was started at the correct weight-based dose for infants less than 1 year of age. Droplet precautions were also initiated. A viral culture from the nasal swab later grew influenza, supporting the result of the rapid test. Clinicians were reluctant to discontinue antibacterial coverage, given the severity of the patient's clinical condition and concern for the risk of bacterial coinfection.

After initiating oseltamivir therapy, the infant continued to require aggressive ventilator support. Because the patient acquired influenza well after his

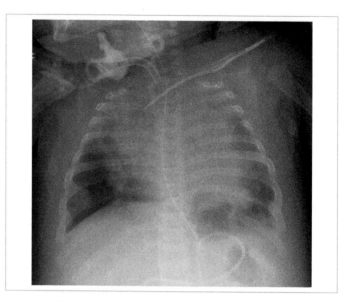

Figure 2.8 Changes of severe chronic lung disease with upper lung zone and parahilar atelectasis, air trapping at the lung bases, and a small left pleural effusion. A tracheostomy tube, central line, and nasogastric tube are also present.

admission to the hospital, the case was considered to be healthcare-associated and the infection control team was notified and a number of interventions were implemented to limit the spread of infection.

Management and Discussion

Although this is a pediatric case, general principles pertaining to influenza-specific laboratory testing, treatment, and prevention apply to the adult population as well. Use of antivirals for treatment of influenza is beyond the scope of this discussion, because emergence of resistant strains has made the selection of an empiric agent more challenging. For example, because of the emergence of resistance to the adamantanes in the last decade, this class is no longer recommended. Therefore, it is important to understand the epidemiology of resistance when selecting empiric therapy, and this is updated continuously by the CDC (http://www.cdc.gov/flu).

To prevent the spread of influenza to other patients in the ward, all patients with suspected or confirmed influenza infection should be placed on droplet precautions according to Healthcare Infection Control Practices Advisory Committee guidelines. Although there has been some controversy concerning the need for N-95 respirators for the protection of healthcare workers especially in the context of the 2009 H1N1 epidemic, available data do not support use of N-95 masks during routine patient care and the CDC currently recommends using airborne precautions only for aerosol-generating procedures including bronchoscopy, sputum induction, endotracheal intubation and extubation, autopsy, cardiopulmonary resuscitation, and open suctioning of airways. Other strategies to prevent spread include placing the patient in a private room or cohorting individuals with laboratory-confirmed influenza together in the same room, minimizing transport from the room unless necessary, and having the patient wear a surgical mask as "source control" to limit the transmission of droplets during sneezing or coughing in the nonventilated patient. Practicing hand hygiene either with soap and water or an alcohol-based hand product before and after every patient encounter is a cornerstone of infection prevention in the hospital that should be emphasized (Tables 2.3 and 2.4).

Table 2.3 Precautions for Prevention of Transmission of Respiratory Infections among Hospitalized Patients

Precautions	Component	Recommendation
Standard	Hand hygiene	Wash hands with soap and water or use an alcohol-based hand rub: before and after contact with a patient; after contact with respiratory secretions; after contact with potentially contaminated items in the patient's vicinity, including equipment and environmental surfaces
	Respiratory hygiene	Instruct staff and visitors with signs and symptoms of a respiratory infection to cover their mouth and nose when sneezing or coughing. Perform hand hygiene after soiling hands with respiratory secretions. Wear masks when tolerated. Maintain spatial separation from others (>0.9 m) when in common waiting areas, if possible
	Gloves	Wear when contact with respiratory secretions could occur
	Gowns	Wear during procedures and activities when contact of clothing or exposed skin with respiratory secretions is anticipated
	Masks and eye protection	Wear during procedures and activities likely to generate splashes or sprays of respiratory secretions
Contact[a]	Patient placement	Place patient in a single-patient room, if possible, or cohort with other patients infected with the same organism
		Limit patient movement to medically necessary purposes
	Gloves and gowns	Wear upon entering room whenever contact is likely with the patient, patient's respiratory secretions, or potentially contaminated items in the patient's vicinity, including equipment and environmental surfaces
	Masks and eye protection	As per standard precautions

Table 2.3 (Continued)		
Precautions	**Component**	**Recommendation**
Droplet[a]	Patient placement	Place patient in a single-patient room, if possible, or cohort with other patients infected with the same organism
		Limit patient movement to medically necessary purposes, and patients should wear a mask and follow respiratory hygiene during transport
	Gloves, gowns, and eye protection	As per standard precautions.
	Masks	Wear a surgical mask on entering room if close contact (eg, <0.9 m) with the patient is anticipated
Airborne[b]	Patient placement	Place infected patients in a single-patient airborne infection isolation room.[b] Patient movement should be limited to medically necessary purposes, and patients should wear a mask and follow respiratory hygiene during transport
	Gloves, gowns, and eye protection	As per standard precautions
	Masks	Wear a fit-tested N95 respirator before room entry

[a] Contact, droplet, and airborne precautions include hand hygiene and respiratory hygiene as per the standard precautions.

[b] Airborne infection isolation room consists of negative pressure relative to the surrounding area and 6 to 12 air changes per hour, and the air is exhausted directly to the outside or recirculated through high-efficiency particulate filtration before return.

Goins WP, Talbot HK, Talbot TR. Health care-acquired viral respiratory diseases. Infect Dis Clin North Am. 2011 Mar;25(1):227–44

In this case, when the parents of the child were asked about recent illnesses among close contacts, the mother stated she had a sore throat a few days earlier. A rapid streptococcal test was positive, and she had received "a shot" from her doctor. Of the 42 HCP with duties in the same area as the patient, 2 reported recent upper respiratory symptoms and 1 reported a recent influenza-like illness (ILI). Several HCP acknowledged working while ill with symptoms. Restriction of ill visitors and HCP is an important strategy for preventing exposure of hospitalized patients to common disease-causing pathogens such as bacteria and viruses from the respiratory tract and skin. Healthcare personnel often report to work despite being ill, putting patients at risk for infection. However in some situations, HCP may be permitted to work as long as certain criteria are met to reduce the risk of disease transmission. For example, at the authors' institution, HCP who have upper respiratory symptoms are

Table 2.4 Pathogen-specific Measures to Prevent the Spread of Viral Respiratory Infections

Infection control recommendations for viral respiratory pathogens

Common measures for reducing transmission in the health care setting

Hand hygiene

Respiratory hygiene/cough etiquette

Standard precautions

Restrict ill visitorsa

Restrict ill personnel for caring for patients at high risk for complications from infection

Cohort nursing

Prompt diagnosis of respiratory infections among patients "by rapid diagnostic testsb

Restrict elective admissions of patients during outbreaks in the community and/or facility

Surveillance for an increase m activity of viral infections within the community

Measures far reducing transmission of specific pathogens in the health care setting

Intervention	RSV	Adenovirus	Parainfluenza Virus	Influenza		
				Seasonal	2009 H1N1	H5N1
Precautions:						
Contact	●	●	●		●	●
Droplet	—	●	—	●	—	—
Airborne	—	—	—	O^c	O^c	●
Eye protection	—	—	—	—	—	●
Vaccination of personnel	—	—	—	●	●	—
Chemoprophylaxis	O^d	—	—	O^e	O^e	●

Closed circles (●) denote recommended measures. Open circles (O) denote measures recommended in certain circumstances.

a Institutions may restrict only young children and or screen all visitors for illness by using a trained health care worker to assess for signs and symptoms or by using an educational patient information list to advise ill visitors.

b To control outbreaks, institutions may perform preadmission screening of patients for infection.

c The CDC recommends health care workers wear respiratory protection such as an N95 respirator during aerosol-generating procedures.

d In addition to other infection control measures, palivizumab prophylaxis of high-risk infants has been used to control outbreaks in the neonatal intensive care unit.

e During a facility outbreak of influenza, administer antiviral chemoprophylaxis to all patients in the involved unit, regardless of the vaccination status, and to unvaccinated personnel working in the involved unit. If feasible, administer facility-wide chemoprophylaxis for all residents in long-term care facilities. Chemoprophylaxis may also be administered to personnel when the outbreak strain is not well matched by the vaccine.

Goins WP, Talbot HK, Talbot TR. Health care-acquired viral respiratory diseases. Infect Dis Clin North Am. 2011 Mar;25(1):227–44.

allowed to work as long as they have been without fever for at least 24 hours and they wear a surgical mask upon entering a patient's room or when working within 3 feet of a patient until symptoms have resolved. Personnel with more severe, influenza-like symptoms may be examined in the institution's employee health service for assessment to determine whether they should be removed from patient care duties. The discussion of the potential for HCP to shed influenza virus in the hospital is made more complex by data suggesting the potential for asymptomatic influenza infection in up to 33% of infected individuals and that influenza virus may be shed up to 1 day before the onset of symptoms. Influenza viral shedding usually abates after resolution of symptoms, but may take up to 10 days to resolve completely.

Antiviral chemoprophylaxis should be considered for family members or other close contacts of a person with suspected or confirmed influenza who are at high risk for influenza complications but have not been vaccinated for the current season. In addition, unvaccinated HCPs who have occupational exposures because of inadequate use of personal protective equipment are candidates for chemoprophylaxis; however, this does not guarantee the individual will not acquire influenza infection or transmit influenza virus.

The most effective way to prevent influenza infection is vaccination. Neither the patient nor either parent had received influenza vaccine for the current season. In the U.S., influenza vaccination coverage among healthy adults historically has been less than 40%. Overall, 13 of the 42 HCP in this case had not been vaccinated, including the HCP with a recent ILI. Children less than 2 years of age and older children with chronic medical conditions are among those groups at greater risk for complications from influenza. Because influenza can also cause severe illness in previously healthy children, the CDC has traditionally recommended vaccination of all children age 6 months to 18 years, adults over age 50, and those in-between with high-risk comorbidities. In 2010, this recommendation was extended to include all persons over 6 months of age regardless of the presence of risk factors (a.k.a. "universal vaccination").

Case Conclusion

The patient became increasingly difficult to ventilate, had worsening cardiac function despite maximal support, and died. Autopsy findings were consistent with influenza viral pneumonia.

Suggested Reading

Bridges CB, Kuehnert MJ, Hall CB. Transmission of influenza: implications for control in health care settings. Clin Infect Dis 2003;37(8):1094–1101.

CDC. Prevention Strategies for Seasonal Influenza in Healthcare Settings. Available at: http://www.cdc.gov/flu/professionals/infectioncontrol/healthcare settings.htm.

Fiore AE, Fry A, Shay D, Gubareva L, Bresee J, Uyeki T; Centers for Disease Control and Prevention (CDC). Antiviral agents for the treatment and chemoprophylaxis of influenza. Recommendations of the Advisory Committee on Immunization Practices (ACIP). MMWR Recomm Rep 2011;60(RR01):1–24.

Fiore AE, Uyeki TM, Broder K, Finelli L, Euler GL, Singleton JA, et al.; Centers for Disease Control and Prevention (CDC). Prevention and control of influenza with vaccines: recommendations of the Advisory Committee on Immunization Practices (ACIP), 2010. MMWR Recomm Rep 2010;59(RR-8):1–62.

Goins WP, Talbot HK, Talbot TR. Health care–acquired viral respiratory diseases. Infect Dis Clin N Am 2011;25:227–244.

Tablan OC, Anderson LJ, Besser R, et al. Guidelines for preventing health-care-associated pneumonia, 2003: recommendations of CDC and the Healthcare Infection Control Practices Advisory Committee. MMWR Recomm Rep 2004;53 (RR-3):1–36.

Talbot HK, Williams JV, Zhu Y, Poehling KA, Griffin MR, Edwards KM. Failure of routine diagnostic methods to detect influenza in hospitalized older adults. Infect Control Hosp Epidemiol 2010l;31(7):683–688.

Chapter 2e

Mycobacterium Tuberculosis

Melanie Gerrior and L.W. Preston Church

Case Presentation and Initial Management

The conclusions and opinions expressed in this chapter are solely the authors' and do not represent the views of the Department of Veterans Affairs or the United States Government.

A 27 year old surgical fellow from Pakistan presents to Pulmonology clinic in her final year of training with wheezing and a dry cough. She first noticed wheezing when she was having difficulty completing her usual 5-km runs. She had no history of night sweats or weight loss. Past medical history included Bacille-Calmette-Guérin (BCG) vaccination as child, a 14-mm Tuberculin Skin Test (TST) 7 years previously and a normal chest radiograph (CXR) on her preemployment physical exam. Since leaving Pakistan she spent a year in Japan followed by internship in Baltimore where she had multiple exposures to *Mycobacterium tuberculosis* (MTB).

Sarcoidosis, tuberculosis, infection due to endemic mycosis, autoimmune lung disease, and hypersensitivity pneumonitis were considered in her differential diagnosis but were all less likely in the setting of a normal CXR. She was diagnosed with asthma, placed on a 6-day oral steroid taper plus inhaled fluticasone/salmeterol and an albuterol rescue inhaler. The cough persisted but she did not seek further medical attention. Three months later she completed fellowship and moved to California. Two weeks after arrival in California her cough steadily increased and she had a fever to 38.5°C. Three sputum samples were smear positive for acid-fast bacilli. She was placed on a four drug regimen consisting of isoniazid (INH), rifampin, ethambutol and pyrazinamide. The infection prevention and control departments of her previous places of employment were notified of her tentative diagnosis.

Discussion

Diagnosis of Latent Tuberculosis

For over 100 years the diagnosis of latent TB has rested on the intradermal injection of purified protein derivative, the TST. Guidelines for interpretation are published and regularly updated by the Centers for Disease Control (Table 2.5). Controversy has surrounded the use of tuberculin skin testing with respect to both sensitivity and specificity, a problem compounded by the lack of a suitable standard of comparison in most situations. Sensitivity is reduced in immunosuppressed individuals, those with active infection, and in the first 8 to 12 weeks after primary infection; in the latter two situations a negative test is never sufficient to exclude infection. False-positive results may be attributed to cross-reactions from exposure to environmental mycobacteria including *Mycobacterium avium-intracellulare* complex and *M. marinum*. The relationship between BCG immunization and the TST is also complex. Administration of BCG in infancy (where it has established benefit) should not contribute to a positive TST after 4 to 5 years. The effect of later BCG administration or boosting is more difficult to assess but may result in a positive TST 10 years later in up to 25% of recipients. In countries where TB is endemic (defined as a prevalence >50/100,000 population), up to 50% of the population is skin test positive—this often proves to be similar to the number of latent infections expected for the burden of active disease (250–500 latent infections for each active case).

Whole-blood interferon gamma release assays (IGRAs) based on the quantification of IFN-γ released by sensitized lymphocytes in response to early secretory antigenic target-6 and culture filtrate protein-10 are an alternative to the TST. These antigens are common to all MTB isolates and pathogenic *M. bovis* strains but not the BCG strain of *M. bovis*. Although a few mycobacteria (*M. szulgai, M. kansasii, M. marinum*) may produce false-positive results, the

Table 2.5 Criteria for a Positive Tuberculin Skin Test

Induration ≥5 mm	Induration ≥10 mm	Induration ≥15 mm
Human immunodeficiency virus (HIV)-positive persons	Residents and employees of high risk settings: health care facilities, prisons and jails, long-term care facilities, homeless shelters, mycobacteriology labs	Persons with no risk factors for TB
Recent contacts of TB case patients	Recent immigrants (within 5 years) from high prevalence countries	
Fibrotic changes on chest radiograph consistent with prior TB	Injection drug users	
Immunosuppression, including organ transplantation, ≥15 mg/day prednisone ≥30 days	Children ≤4 years of age or ≤18 years of age and exposed to adults at high risk	
	Other conditions associated with increased risk of disease, including silicosis, diabetes mellitus, chronic renal failure, leukemias and lymphomas, lung cancer, head and neck cancer, weight loss ≥10% of ideal body weight, gastrectomy, jejunoileal bypass	

Adapted from: CDC. Targeted tuberculin testing and treatment of latent tuberculosis infection. MMWR 2000;49(RR-6):1–51.

Table 2.6 Comparison of TST and IGRAs in Predicting Risk of Progression to Active Tuberculosis		
	TST	**IGRA**
Sensitivity	90%–100%	80%–90%
Specificity	29%–39%	56%–83%
Positive Predictive Value	2.7%–3.1%	4%–8%
Negative Predictive Value	99%–100%	99%–100%

Pooled results from 4 published studies examining household contacts of an active TB case. Positive TST defined as a reaction >5 mm induration.

specificity of IGRAs is superior to that of the TST. Although the sensitivity of these assays may be slightly less than the TST, the ability to identify individuals at risk for progression to active TB appears to be similar (Table 2.6). Guidelines for the use of IGRAs have been published. Issues of cost effectiveness and managing discordant IGRAs and TST remain unsettled.

Contact Investigation

Nosocomial transmission of MTB is rarely encountered in the United States in the twenty-first century. Transmission risk is multidirectional and prevention efforts must consider the possibilities of patient-to-patient, patient-to-health-care worker (HCW) and HCW-to-patient transmission. Recognizing potential cases of active tuberculosis, employing appropriate negative pressure isolation and the use of fit-tested N95 or equivalent respiratory protection by HCWs are essential to minimizing the risk in the first two scenarios.

The last rotation for the surgery fellow prior to completion of fellowship was the pediatric intensive care unit. In conjunction with occupational and employee health, the infection prevention and control team generated a contact list of patients and staff who were potentially exposed while in the unit over the time period corresponding to the fellow's rotation schedule and history of symptoms. The list of HCW included nurses, physicians, respiratory therapists, physical therapists, as well as ancillary staff. All exposed staff were offered immediate and 3-month TST. Parents were notified and all children cared for in the unit during that time were administered a TST. No child had a positive TST.

Defining a contact and stratifying the risk of infection is dependent on several variables, including the disease characteristics of the source; the age and immune status of the contact; the presence of comorbid illness in the contact; the physical characteristics of the space where contact occurred (size, ventilation); and the duration, intensity, and distance between the source and the contact. Defining the level of risk posed by the source is challenging because the factors influencing transmission of MTB remain incompletely understood. Cough and type of disease (cavitary, lung, laryngeal, endobronchial) are important and the level of smear positivity may serve as a rough surrogate of infectivity, although there is individual variability in the effectiveness of transmission and a considerable burden of infection is transmitted by smear negative cases. Consequently any contact of an infected HCW requires education and evaluation, including TST. This process is stratified by risk, addressing contacts at greatest risk of infection and disease first. As a general rule contact tracing should reach back 3 months from the time of diagnosis of the index case, but this varies according to the circumstances. Early after exposure the initial TST serves as a baseline or to identify individuals positive by previous exposure, with a follow up TST 12 weeks after exposure as a screen for new infection. Under most circumstances this is a sufficient and safe practice. For exposed individuals at high risk of rapidly emerging disease, including children under 5 and immunocompromised patients, it may be prudent to initiate single drug therapy (usually INH) pending the results of a TST at 12 weeks.

When may the infected HCW return to patient care duties? The answer will vary by facility and generally will be recommended in collaboration with the infection prevention and control and employee/occupational health teams. Data to support any position is scant but it is well demonstrated that viable MTB can persist in expectorated sputum for weeks or months after initiation of appropriate therapy. A conservative approach would be to restrict the HCW from patient contact until consistently negative smears are collected and a minimum of 2 weeks of effective therapy has been completed.

Case Presentation (continued)

Could this case have been prevented? Managing the positive TST in a HCW remains a contentious subject. Although risk of reactivation is greatest in the first 2 years after infection, this case demonstrates that a finite risk exists even after this period (if the TST was a true positive) and other factors may intervene which enhance this risk. Conversely, individuals with a positive TST may believe they are "'immune'" and fail to utilize personal protective gear, placing them at risk for acquisition of new infection. Single drug therapy for latent TB does carry some risk and is at best only 90% effective; this risk for the

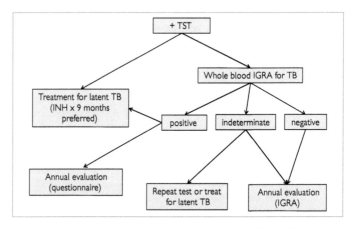

Figure 2.9 Management Algorithm for the Tuberculin Skin Test-Positive Healthcare Worker. *Solid arrows* represent preferred pathways, *dashed arrows* represent alternative pathways for individuals declining treatment.

practicing HCW, however, remains lower than the risk of reactivation of latent TB detected at any time point after infection. All newly TST positive HCW should be encouraged to take INH for a period of 9 months (or weekly INH + rifapentene × 12 weeks based on recently concluded clinical trails); those declining or known to have previous BCG immunization or positive TST should have an IGRA and be managed as outlined in Figure 2.9.

Case Conclusion

The surgeon was treated with INH, rifampin, ethambutol, and pyrazinamide as directly observed therapy by the local health department. She had converted to smear negative by the third week and her isolate was susceptible to all first-line agents. At the end of 8 weeks her regimen was reduced to INH and rifampin three times weekly and she completed a total of 24 weeks of therapy.

Suggested Reading

CDC. Guidelines for the investigation of contacts of persons with infectious tuberculosis. MMWR 2005;54(RR-15):1–47.

CDC. Guidelines for preventing the transmission of *Mycobacterium tuberculosis* in health-care settings, 2005. MMWR 2005;54(RR-17):1–140.

CDC. Mycobacterium tuberculosis transmission in a newborn nursery and maternity ward—New York City, 2003. MMWR 2005;54:1280–1283.

CDC. Targeted tuberculin testing and treatment of latent tuberculosis infection. MMWR 2000;49(RR-6):1–51.

CDC. Updated guidelines for using interferon gamma release assays to detect *Mycobacterium tuberculosis* infection - United States, 2010. MMWR 2010;59 (RR-5):1–25.

Horsburgh CR, Rubin EJ. Latent tuberculosis infection in the United States. NEJM 2011;364:1441–1448.

Mazurek GH, Zajdowicz MJ, Hankinson AL, Costigan DJ, Toney SR, Rothel JS, et al. Detection of *Mycobacterium tuberculosis* infection in United States Navy recruits using the tuberculin skin test or whole-blood interferon-γ release assays. Clin Infect Dis 2007;45:826–836.

Chapter 3a

Central Line-Associated Bloodstream Infection

David B. Banach and David P. Calfee

Case Presentation

A 41-year old male with a history of orthotopic heart transplantation for dilated cardiomyopathy presents to the emergency department (ED) with 3 days of progressive cough, orthopnea, and paroxysmal nocturnal dyspnea. In the ED he is afebrile but is mildly hypoxic and requires supplemental oxygen through a simple facemask. Cardiac examination reveals an S3 gallop and marked jugular venous distension. Pulmonary auscultation reveals bilateral inspiratory crackles extending to the lung apices.

He is diagnosed with congestive heart failure, attributed to cellular rejection of the transplanted heart. His symptoms of volume overload do not improve with diuresis so, while still in the ED, a central venous catheter is placed in the left internal jugular vein for hemodynamic monitoring and administration of vasodilator and inotropic medications. He is then admitted to the cardiology service for further management.

On the seventh day of hospitalization he is febrile (39.1° C) and his heart rate is 116 beats per minute. Examination of the central venous catheter insertion site reveals mild erythema but no drainage or fluctuance. There are no other signs of infection identified during a thorough physical examination. Laboratory studies reveal leukocytosis. Two sets of blood cultures are obtained by peripheral venipuncture at two separate sites.

Differential Diagnosis and Initial Management

Central line-associated bloodstream infections (CLABSI) are a major cause of morbidity and mortality among hospitalized patients and are associated with substantial cost to the healthcare system. Although most attention towards CLABSI has focused on intensive care units (ICUs), there is an increasing awareness of these infections in non-ICU settings. In fact, in U.S. hospitals, the majority of CLABSI occur outside of the ICU. Asymptomatic bacterial or fungal colonization or contamination of the catheter typically precedes a catheter-related bloodstream infection. Microorganisms may colonize the extraluminal catheter surface, most frequently because of contamination during insertion or migration of bacteria present on the skin at the insertion site, or the intraluminal surface, because of contamination of the catheter hub or tubing during use, or rarely, infected intravenous fluids. The diagnosis of CLABSI should be considered in any patient with an intravascular catheter and fever and/or other signs of systemic infection. Although the presence of inflammation or purulence at the catheter site is frequently absent, the vascular catheter and associated exit site and tract should be thoroughly examined, and any inflammatory signs should prompt consideration of catheter removal. Any positive blood culture in a patient with a central venous catheter should raise the suspicion for CLABSI.

Epidemiologically, a CLABSI is defined as a bloodstream infection in a patient with a central venous catheter in place at the time of or within 48 hours of collection of the blood sample, for which no other source of the bloodstream infection (e.g., pneumonia, surgical site infection) can be identified. A definitive clinical diagnosis of catheter-related bloodstream infection requires that the same organism grow from at least one percutaneous blood sample and a catheter source culture, which may consist of catheter-aspirated blood or a catheter tip segment culture if the catheter is removed. These definitions may guide clinicians in the diagnosis of CLABSI in various clinical settings. Although blood cultures drawn solely from central venous catheters are highly sensitive for the detection of CLABSI, they are of lower specificity than cultures from peripheral veins.

In a suspected CLABSI, blood cultures should be obtained before the initiation of antibiotic therapy. Blood cultures should be drawn from two separate sites. At least one of these sets of blood cultures should be obtained from a peripheral vein by percutaneous venipuncture. The sensitivity of blood cultures is highly dependent on specimen quantity, and 30 to 40 ml provides optimal sensitivity. In routine clinical practice 10 ml of blood is obtained per culture site. Quantitative blood cultures or differential time to positivity (DTP) of paired blood cultures drawn from a catheter and peripherally may be useful in establishing the catheter as the source of bloodstream infection, particularly among long-term catheters. A microbial colony count from a catheter culture specimen of over threefold greater than the colony count from a peripheral blood culture is suggestive of a CLABSI. For DTP, CLABSI is suggested by detection of growth of microbes from blood drawn from a catheter at least 2 hours before growth is detected in a simultaneously drawn peripheral blood culture.

The case presented here, fever and tachycardia in a patient with a central venous catheter, prompts evaluation of the catheter site revealing erythema, which may be suggestive of a catheter-related infection.

Case Presentation (Continued)

Based on the epidemiology of the suspected pathogens associated with CLABSI, empiric antibiotic therapy with vancomycin and cefepime is initiated. Within 12 hours, the laboratory reports that both sets of blood cultures are positive for gram positive cocci in clusters. The clinician decides that the central venous catheter will be removed. The following day, the organism isolated from the blood cultures is identified as methicillin-susceptible *Staphylococcus aureus*. Vancomycin and cefepime are discontinued and cefazolin is begun.

Management

Following the obtainment of blood cultures, empiric antibiotic therapy is initiated. Factors that influence the choice of antibiotic therapy include the severity of illness, the suspected pathogens associated with the CLABSI, and local antibiotic susceptibility patterns. Previous microbiological test results for the patient, when available, should also be considered during the selection of empiric antimicrobial therapy. Most CLABSI are caused by coagulase-negative staphylococci and *Staphylococcus aureus*, both of which are often resistant to methicillin, followed by gram-negative organisms and *Candida* species. Until additional culture data is available it is reasonable to initiate empiric therapy with broad spectrum antibiotics. The decision to add empirical coverage for gram-negative bacilli and fungal pathogens, and the selection of specific empiric antimicrobial therapy targeting these organisms, should be based on local epidemiology and antimicrobial susceptibility patterns, the location of the catheter, the patient's underlying risk factors, and the severity of illness. Empiric antibiotic therapy should be adjusted based on blood culture results, once available. Decisions regarding the duration of antibiotic therapy in treating CLABSI are dependent on the causative organism, the time until bacterial or fungal clearance, and the presence of secondary complications of infection including sepsis and metastatic seeding of infection. Figures 3.1 and 3.2 provide detailed guidance addressing the selection of antimicrobial therapy, duration of therapy, and catheter removal in the management of short-term and long-term catheters, including totally implanted devices (e.g., ports). Guidelines by the Infectious Diseases Society of America published in 2009 provide evidence-based recommendations and a detailed review of the diagnosis and treatment of vascular catheter-related infections.

The decision regarding catheter removal is an essential component of the management of CLABSI. The causative pathogen, catheter type, location of the catheter, and severity of illness should be considered when making decisions regarding catheter removal. Long-term catheters should be removed in cases of severe illness (e.g., sepsis), persistent bloodstream infection despite appropriate antibiotic therapy, infection of the catheter tunnel tract, or secondary infection such as endocarditis, suppurative thrombophlebitis, or osteomyelitis. The isolation of *Staphylococcus aureus* or *Candida* species as the source of CLABSI should also prompt the decision to remove a long-term central venous catheter in most cases. For uncomplicated infections caused by organisms such as coagulase-negative staphylococci, *Enterococcus*, and gram-negative bacilli, catheter salvage can be considered in conjunction with systemic antibiotics and antibiotic lock therapy. In general, temporary, nontunneled catheters should be removed in the setting of CLABSI, although catheter salvage may be considered in some patients with infections due to coagulase-negative staphylococci.

Evidence-based recommendations for the prevention of CLABSI primarily focus on minimizing the risk of catheter contamination during catheter insertion, use, and maintenance (Table 3.1). Healthcare worker education regarding proper techniques for catheter insertion, use, and maintenance, the use of maximal sterile barrier precautions during catheter insertion, the use of 2% chlorhexidine solution for skin antisepsis, and prompt removal of central venous catheters as soon as they are no longer needed are all recommended.

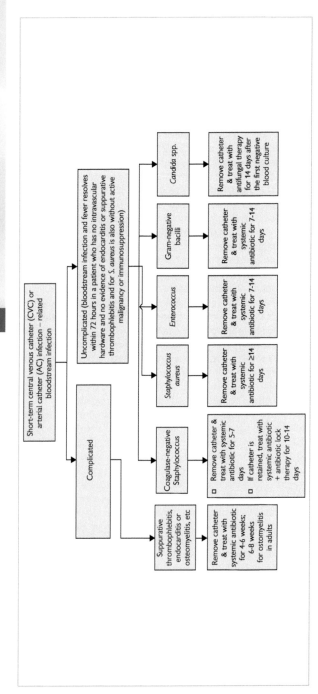

Figure 3.1 Approach to the management of patients with short-term central venous catheter-related bloodstream infection.

(From Mermel LA, Allon M, Bouza E, et al. Clinical practice guidelines for the diagnosis and management of intravascular catheter-related infection: 2009 update by the Infectious Diseases Society of America. Clin Infect Dis 2009;49:1–45. Used with permission from Oxford University Press and the Infectious Diseases Society of America.)

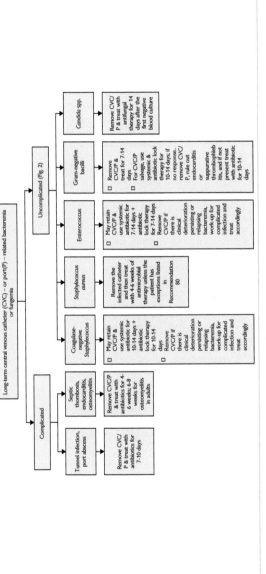

Long-term central venous catheter (CVC) – or port(P) – related bacteremia or fungemia

Complicated

- Tunnel infection, port abscess
  - Remove CVC/P & treat with antibiotics for 7-10 days
- Septic thrombosis, endocarditis, osteomyelitis
  - Remove CVC/P & treat with antibiotics for 4-6 weeks; 6-8 weeks for osteomyelitis in adults

Uncomplicated (Fig. 2)

- Coagulase-negative Staphylococcus
  - ☐ May retain CVC/P & use systemic antibiotic for 10-14 days + antibiotic lock therapy for 10-14 days
  - ☐ Remove CVC/P if there is clinical deterioration persisting or relapsing bacteremia, work-up for complicated infection and treat accordingly

- Staphylococcus aureus
  - Remove the infected catheter and then treat with 4-6 weeks of antimicrobial therapy unless the patient has exceptions listed in Recommendation 80

- Enterococcus
  - ☐ May retain CVC/P & use systemic & lock therapy for 7-14 days + antibiotic lock therapy for 7-14 days
  - ☐ Remove CVC/P if there is clinical deterioration persisting or relapsing bacteremia, work-up for complicated infection and treat accordingly

- Gram-negative bacilli
  - ☐ Remove CVC/P & treat for 7-14 days
  - ☐ For CVC/P salvage, use systemic & antibiotic lock therapy for 10-14 days; if no response, remove CVC/P, rule out endocarditis or suppurative thrombophlebitis, and if not present treat with antibiotic for 10-14 days

- Candida spp.
  - Remove CVC/P & treat with antifungal therapy for 14 days after the first negative blood culture

Figure 3.2 Approach to the Management of Patients with Long-Term Central Venous Catheter-Related Bloodstream Infection

Uncomplicated: bloodstream infection and fever resolves within 72 hours in a patient who has no intravascular hardware and no evidence of endocarditis or suppurative thrombophlebitis and for *Staphylococcus aureus* is also without active malignancy or immunosuppression.

Recommendation 80: Patients can be considered for a shorter duration of antimicrobial therapy (i.e., a minimum of 14 days of therapy) if the patient is not diabetic; if the patient is not immunosuppressed; if the infected catheter is removed; if the patient has no prosthetic intravascular device; if there is no evidence of endocarditis or suppurative thrombophlebitis on TEE and ultrasound, respectively; if fever and bacteremia resolve within 72 hours after initiation of appropriate antimicrobial therapy; and if there is no evidence of metastatic infection on physical examination and sign- or symptom-directed diagnostic tests.

(From Mermel LA, Allon M, Bouza E, et al. Clinical practice guidelines for the diagnosis and management of intravascular catheter-related infection: 2009 update by the Infectious Diseases Society of America. Clin Infect Dis 2009;49:1–45. Used with permission from Oxford University Press and the Infectious Diseases Society of America.)

Table 3.1 Strategies for the Prevention of Central Line-Associated Bloodstream Infections

Strategy	Comment
Healthcare worker (HCW) education	Educate HCWs regarding proper catheter insertion, use and maintenance techniques.
	Periodically assess the knowledge and skills of all persons involved in catheter insertion, use and maintenance.
Hand hygiene	Hand hygiene must be performed before catheter insertion and before catheter use or manipulation.
	Hand washing with conventional antiseptic containing soap and water or waterless alcohol based foams or gels is recommended.
Catheter site selection	The subclavian site has been associated with the lowest rate of infectious complications. The femoral site has been associated with the highest rate of infectious complications, and should be avoided when possible.
Catheter insertion	A sterile gown and gloves and a non-sterile cap and mask should be worn by all individuals involved in central venous catheter insertion, and the patient should be covered in a sterile drape during insertion.
	Although 2% chlorhexidine gluconate is the preferred agent for skin antisepsis for patients older than 2 months of age, tincture of iodine, an iodophor, or 70% alcohol are acceptable.
Catheter maintenance and use	Gauze dressings should be changed every other day, or if they become loose, damp or visibly soiled.
	Transparent dressings should be changed at least every 7 days or if they become loose, damp, or visibly soiled.
	Clean injection ports with chlorhexidine, 70% alcohol, or an iodophor with friction prior to accessing the catheter.
	Assess central venous catheter necessity daily and remove any catheter that is no longer necessary.
Other preventive measures that may be useful	Daily bathing of patients with chlorhexidine gluconate has been associated with a reduced incidence of CLABSI in long-term care facilities and intensive care units.
	Antibiotic or antiseptic impregnated catheters have been associated, in some studies, with a reduced incidence of CLABSI.
	The use of chlorhexidine-impregnated dressings at the catheter exit site has been associated with reduced rates of CLABSI.

Case Conclusion

The central venous catheter, a short-term catheter, was removed. The patient's fever resolved and subsequent blood cultures obtained 24 hours after catheter removal were sterile. A transesophageal echocardiogram was performed and revealed no evidence of valvular vegetations. Cefazolin was continued to complete a 28-day course.

Suggested Reading

Burton D, Edwards J, Horan T, Jernigan J, Fridkin S. Methicillin-resistant *Staphylococcus aureus* central line-associated bloodstream infections in US intensive care units, 1997–2007. JAMA 2009;301:727–736.

Maki DG, Kluger DM, Crnich CJ. The risk of bloodstream infection in adults with different intravascular devices: a systematic review of 200 published prospective studies. Mayo Clin Proc 2006;81:1159–1171.

Mermel L, Allon M, Bouza E, Craven D, Flynn P, O'Grady N, et al. Clinical practice guidelines for the diagnosis and management of intravascular catheter-related infection: 2009 Update by the Infectious Diseases Society of America. Clin Infect Dis 2009;49:1–45.

O'Grady NP, Alexander M, Burns LA, Dellinger EP, Garland J, Heard SO, et al.; Healthcare Infection Control Practices Advisory Committee. Guidelines for the prevention of intravascular catheter-related infections, 2011. Clin Infect Dis 2011;52(9):1087–1099.

Wisplinghoff H, Bischoff T, Tallent S, Seifert H, Wenzel R, Edmond M. Nosocomial bloodstream infections in US hospitals: analysis of 24,179 cases from a prospective nationwide surveillance study. Clin Infect Dis 2004;39:309–317.

Chapter 3b

Staphylococcus aureus Bacteremia and Endocarditis

Aimee Hodowanec and Kyle J. Popovich

Case Presentation

A 35-year-old woman with a history of short gut syndrome following surgical management of severe Crohn's disease presented to the emergency department (ED) reporting 2 days of subjective fevers and general malaise. Upon arrival in the ED, the patient is found to be febrile to 38.9° C, tachycardic (110 beats per minute), and normotensive (128/80 mm Hg). She has a right upper extremity peripherally inserted central catheter (PICC) in place, through which she receives home total parenteral nutrition. Examination of the surrounding skin reveals no tenderness, erythema, or purulent drainage. Her abdomen is soft and nontender. Blood cultures are obtained from the catheter and percutaneously. She is given intravenous fluids and started on broad spectrum antibiotics.

Differential Diagnosis and Initial Management

Fever in a patient with an indwelling vascular catheter should elicit a strong suspicion for a bloodstream infection. Both methicillin-susceptible S aureus (MSSA) and methicillin resistant S aureus (MRSA) are common causes of bloodstream infections in adults.[1] The presence of an intravascular catheter is a significant risk factor for a staphylococcal bloodstream infection. Additional specific risk factors for methicillin-resistant infections include the presence of percutaneous devices, recent hospitalization or surgery, residence in a long-term care facility, and renal disease requiring hemodialysis.[2]

There are several methods used for classifying S aureus bloodstream infections. The infection is generally considered nosocomial if more than 48 hours elapse between hospital admission and bloodstream infection. Healthcare-associated bacteremia can be defined as occurring in the outpatient setting or within 48 hours of hospital admission in a patient meeting at least one of the following criteria: presence of an invasive device at the time of admission; history of MRSA infection or colonization; or history of surgery, hospitalization, dialysis or residence in a long-term care facility in the preceding 12 months.

Community-associated bloodstream infections can be classified as those that occur in the outpatient setting or within 48 hours of hospitalization in a patient who does not otherwise meet criteria for healthcare associated infection.[3] Additionally, S. aureus bacteremia can be described as complicated or uncomplicated. To be considered uncomplicated, the following criteria must be met: no evidence of endocarditis, no implanted prosthesis, negative follow-up blood cultures obtained 2 to 4 days after initial cultures, resolution of fever within 72 hours of initiating effective antimicrobial therapy, and no evidence of metastatic infection.[4] S. aureus bloodstream infections not meeting these criteria are considered complicated. These epidemiologic and clinical categorizations impact both the prevention and treatment of S. aureus bloodstream infections.

S. aureus bacteremia is associated with significant morbidity and mortality. Fowler et al. observed that of patients with S. aureus bacteremia (MSSA or MRSA), 34% of patients developed metastatic infection (such as prosthetic device infection, septic arthritis, deep tissue abscess, vertebral osteomyelitis, epidural abscess, psoas abscess, or meningitis), 12% had confirmed endocarditis, and 22% died.[5] Therefore, prompt diagnosis with timely initiation of appropriate therapy is essential. Proper technique for the collection of blood cultures is critical for making the diagnosis of a bloodstream infection. According to the 2009 Infectious Diseases Society of America (IDSA) guidelines, the skin and catheter hubs should be prepared with alcohol, tincture of iodine, or alcoholic chlorhexidine (10.5%) and patients should have at least 2 sets of blood cultures collected prior to the initiation of antimicrobial therapy. If an indwelling catheter is present, cultures should be obtained from the catheter as well as percutaneously. For multilumen catheters, the utility of culturing each lumen remains unclear.[6] If a patient is hemodynamically unstable or if there is a strong clinical suspicion for a bloodstream infection, empiric antimicrobial therapy should be initiated while awaiting culture results.[6]

Given the high incidence of infective endocarditis, every patient with S. aureus bloodstream infection should undergo echocardiography.[4] Transesophageal echocardiography (TEE) is preferred over transthoracic echocardiography (TTE) in this setting as it is more sensitive for detecting valvular lesions. Shively et al. found that the sensitivity and specificity of a TEE is 94% and 100%, respectively. Comparatively, a TTE has a sensitivity of only 44% and a specificity of 98%.[7] One study observed that the sensitivity of a TEE is further increased when the test is performed at least 5 to 7 days after onset of bacteremia.[6]

Case Presentation (continued)

Later on the day of admission, the Gram stain from the patient's blood culture shows gram-positive cocci in clusters. That night, she has an episode of rigors and is again noted to be febrile. The following day blood cultures are reported to be growing S. aureus, which is ultimately identified as MRSA. A transesophageal echocardiogram is obtained and reveals a large, mobile vegetation on the mitral valve. Trace mitral regurgitation is noted as well. However, the patient remains hemodynamically stable, without evidence of metastatic infection. All antimicrobial agents except for vancomycin are discontinued. Her PICC is promptly removed.

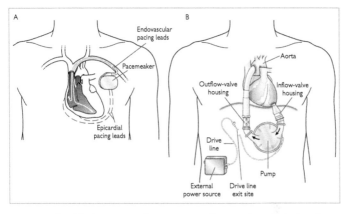

Figure 3.3 Panel **A** demonstrates the components of a pacemaker, with both endovascular leads (*solid lines*) and epicardial leads (*dashed lines*). Panel **B** demonstrates the
components of an LVAD.

Management

An increasing proportion of S aureus infections are caused by MRSA. In 2003,
64.4% of hospital-onset S. aureus infections in U.S. intensive care units were
caused by MRSA.[8] In the 2011 IDSA guidelines for the treatment of MRSA infections, intravenous vancomycin is the recommended therapy for the treatment
of MRSA bacteremia. Potential concerns with vancomycin therapy include drug
toxicity (such as nephrotoxicity and high-frequency hearing loss associated with
high serum trough levels),[4] requirement for monitoring of trough drug levels to
ensure safe and effective dosing, and the possible increase in the vancomycin
minimum inhibitory concentration that has been reported at several centers
(so-called "MIC creep"). Because of increasing reports of treatment failure
when vancomycin is used to treat MRSA isolates with borderline or interme-
diate susceptibility to the drug, the Clinical and Laboratory Standards Institute
reevaluated vancomycin MIC breakpoints and ultimately lowered them in 2006
(Table 3.2).[4] Among vancomycin susceptible (MIC ≤2.0) S. aureus strains, the
MIC has been reported to "creep" up and approach the 2 µg/ml breakpoint
among patients on therapy with increasing frequency over the past decade.[9]
Although the significance of this shift is unclear, a recent study did find that
vancomycin MICs of 1.0 to 2.0 may be associated with higher rates of MRSA
bacteremia treatment failure when compared with more susceptible isolates.[10]
However, the IDSA MRSA guidelines currently recommend that for isolates
with an MIC of 2.0 µg/ml or greater, the patient's clinical response should be
followed to determine if vancomycin can be used, irrespective of the MIC.[4] In
patients who cannot tolerate vancomycin or who appear to not be responding
to treatment, daptomycin is an alternative agent with bactericidal activity. In a
study by Fowler et al, daptomycin was found not to be inferior to vancomycin

for the treatment of both *S aureus* (MSSA and MRSA) bacteremia and right-sided endocarditis.[11]

Bloodstream MRSA infections complicated by endocarditis require special therapeutic consideration. For treatment of native-valve endocarditis, there are conflicting data regarding the clinical benefit of combination therapy with an aminoglycoside added to vancomycin. Although earlier studies suggested a role for aminoglycoside therapy, a study by Cosgrove, et al. demonstrated increased nephrotoxicity with the addition of aminoglycosides.[12] The 2005 American Heart Association endocarditis guidelines state that the use of aminoglycosides can be considered for the treatment of native valve endocarditis, but the use should be limited to the first 3 to 5 days of treatment.[13] More recently, the 2011 IDSA MRSA guidelines recommend that aminoglycosides not be used in the treatment of *S. aureus* native valve endocarditis.[4] In contrast, in the case of prosthetic-valve endocarditis, combination therapy is recommended. In addition to vancomycin, patients should receive rifampin for the duration of therapy as well as an aminoglycoside (gentamicin) for the first 2 weeks of therapy.[13] All patients with MRSA prosthetic valve endocarditis should undergo prompt evaluation for possible valve replacement or repair.[13]

In cases of MSSA bacteremia and endocarditis, a semisynthetic penicillin such as nafcillin or oxacillin, is the recommended therapy.[13] The only exception to this guidance is for patients with a documented anaphylactic penicillin allergy, for whom vancomycin is recommended. Semisynthetic penicillins and first-generation cephalosporins appear to have better activity than vancomycin for the treatment of MSSA. Nafcillin has been associated with shorter time to resolution of MSSA bacteremia (with or without endocarditis) and less frequent relapse of infection compared to treatment with vancomycin.[14] Among hemodialysis patients with complicated or uncomplicated MSSA bacteremia, vancomycin has been associated with an increased risk of treatment failure (defined as death or recurrent infection) as compared with cefazolin.[15] Therefore, in the absence of a severe β-lactam allergy, vancomycin generally should not be used for the treatment of MSSA bloodstream infections. The management of MSSA endocarditis is similar to MRSA endocarditis. The addition of an aminoglycoside is primarily reserved for prosthetic-valve endocarditis and timely surgical evaluation is again essential.

Determining the appropriate duration of therapy for an *S. aureus* bloodstream infection can be challenging. The clinical classifications schemes described (Table 3.3) can provide guidance in determining treatment duration. In adults

Table 3.2 2006 Revised CLSI Vancomycin MIC Breakpoints for *S aureus*

S aureus Classification	MIC Breakpoint
Vancomycin susceptible *S aureus*	≤ 2.0 µg/ml
Vancomycin intermediate *S aureus* (VISA)	$4.0 - 8.0$ µg/ml
Vancomycin resistant *S aureus* (VRSA)	≥ 16.0 µg/ml
CLSI, Clinical and Laboratory Standards Institute; MIC, minimum inhibitory concentration.	

Table 3.3 Therapy for *Staphylococcus aureus* Bloodstream Infections

Type of Infection	Organism	Preferred Antimicrobial Agent	Alternative Antimicrobial Agent	Duration (Weeks)	Comment
Uncomplicated Bacteremia	Methicillin-susceptible strains	Nafcillin or oxacillin 12 g/24 h IV in 4–6 equally divided doses	Cefazolin 6g/24 h IV in 3 equally divided doses	≥2	Bacteremia is considered uncomplicated if: no evidence of endocarditis, no implanted prosthesis, negative follow up blood cultures obtained 2–4 days after initial cultures, defervescense within 72 hours of initiating effective antimicrobial therapy, and no evidence of metastatic infection.
	Methicillin-resistant strains	Vancomycin 15–20 mg/kg/dose IV every 8–12 h[a]	Daptomycin 6mg/kg IV every 24 h	≥2	
Complicated Bacteremia	Methicillin-susceptible strains	Nafcillin or oxacillin 12 g/24 h IV in 4–6 equally divided doses	Cefazolin 6g/24 h IV in 3 equally divided doses	4–6[c]	For native valve *S. aureus* endocarditis, combination therapy with aminoglycosides is not routinely recommended. For prosthetic valve *S. aureus* endocarditis, gentamicin 1mg/kg IV every 8 h and rifampin 300mg PO/IV every 8 h should be added to the regimen.[b]
	Methicillin-resistant strains	Vancomycin 15–20 mg/kg/dose IV every 8–12 h[a]	Daptomycin 6mg/kg IV every 24 h	4–6[c]	

IV, intravenous; PO, oral

[a] Adjust vancomycin dose to attain trough level of 15–20 μg/mL

[b] Gentamicin should be administered for first 2 weeks of therapy and rifampin for duration of therapy.

[c] *S. aureus* endocarditis is treated for 6 weeks (with the exception of uncomplicated, right-sided MSSA endocarditis which can be treated for 2 weeks).

with uncomplicated bacteremia (as previously defined), at least 2 weeks of intravenous antibiotics should be administered. For complicated bacteremia, 4 to 6 weeks of therapy is recommended.[4] For patients with infective endocarditis, a 6 week course of therapy is recommended. The exception to this is patients with uncomplicated, right-sided endocarditis caused by MSSA. In this setting, a 2-week course of combined β-lactam and aminoglycoside may be sufficient.[13]

Catheter-related bloodstream infections (CRBSI) also deserve special consideration. The 2009 IDSA guidelines on the management of intravascular catheter-related infections recommend that all patients with *S. aureus* CRBSI have their catheter removed, regardless if whether it is a long- or short-term catheter. The guidelines also recommend that the majority of patients with *S. aureus* CRBSI receive 4 to 6 weeks of therapy.[6] A shorter duration (at least 2 weeks) may be considered if the patient is not diabetic; not immunosuppressed; the catheter is removed; there is no prosthetic intravascular device; there is no evidence of suppurative thrombophlebitis, endocarditis, or metastatic infection; and the fever and bacteremia resolve within 72 hours of initiating appropriate antimicrobial therapy.[6]

The significant morbidity and mortality as well as high cost associated with treating bloodstream infections make preventing such infections a priority. In 2011, IDSA published updated guidelines for the prevention of catheter-related infections. Recommendations cited in these guidelines include: improved education on intravascular catheter insertion and use; use of an upper-extremity site for catheter insertion; use of aseptic technique for insertion of the catheter; hand hygiene before manipulation or assessment of the catheter; evaluation of the insertion site daily for signs of infection; replacement of dressing on the catheter every 2 to 7 days depending on catheter and dressing type; and removal of the catheter if it malfunctions, is no longer necessary, or if signs of infection are present.[16]

Case Conclusion

The most likely source of MRSA in this patient is her PICC. Following removal of the catheter, no additional blood cultures were positive. She was evaluated by cardiothoracic surgery, but no surgical intervention was found to be necessary. A new PICC was placed after additional blood cultures demonstrated no growth. She had an uneventful hospital course and is discharged home to receive 6 weeks of vancomycin.

References

Friedman ND, Kaye KS, Stout JE, et al. Health care-associated bloodstream infections in adults: a reason to change the accepted definition of community-acquired infections. Ann Intern Med 2002;137:791–797.

Naimi TS, LeDell KH, Como-Sabetti K, et al. Comparison of community and health care-associated methecillin-resistant *Staphylococcus aureus* infection. J Am Med Assoc 2003;290:2976–2984.

Klevens RM, Morrison MA, Nadle J, et al. Invasive methicillin-resistant *Staphylococcus aureus* infections in the United States. J Am Med Assoc 2007;298:1763–1771.

Liu C, Bayer A, Cosgrove S, et al. Clinical practice guidelines by the infectious disease society of America for the treatment of methicillin-resistant *Staphylococcus aureus* infections in adults and children. Clin Infect Dis 2011;52:1–38.

Fowler VG Jr, Olsen MK, Corey GR, et al. Clinical identifiers of complicated *Staphylococcus aureus* bactermia. Arch Intern Med 2003:163: 2066–2072.

Mermel L, Allon M, Bouza E, et al. Clinical practice guidelines for the diagnosis and management of intravascular catheter-related infection: 2009 update by the infectious diseases society of America. Clin Infect Dis 2009;49:1–45.

Shively BK, Gurule FT, Roldan CA, Leggett JH, Schiller NB. Diagnostic value of transesophageal compared with transthoracic echocardiography in infective endocarditis. J Am Coll Cardiol 1991;18:391–397.

Klevens RM, Edwards JR, Tenover FC, McDonald LC, Horan T, Gaynes R. Changes in the epidemiology of methicillin-resistant *Staphylococcus aureus* in intensive care units in U.S. hospitals, 1992–2003. Clin Infect Dis 2006;42:389–391.

Wang G, Hindler JF, Ward KW, et al. Increased vancomycin MICs for Staphylococcus aureus clinical isolates from a university hospital during a 5-year period. J Clin Microbiol 2006;44:3883–3886.

Sakoulas G, Moise-Broder PA, Schentag J, et al. Relationship of MIC and bactericidal activity to efficacy of vancomycin for treatment of methicillin-resistant *Staphylococcus aureus* bactermia. J Clin Microbiol 2004;42(6):2398–2402.

Fowler VG Jr, Boucher HW, Corey GR, et al. Daptomycin versus standard therapy for bactermia and endocarditis caused by *Staphylococcus aureus*. NEJM 2006;355:653–655.

Cosgrove SE, Vigliani GA, Fowler VG, et al. Initial low-dose gentamicin for *Staphylococcus aureus* bacteremia and endocarditis is nephrotoxic. Clin Infect Dis 2009; 48:713–721.

Baddour L, Wilson W, Bayer A, et al. Infective endocarditis: diagnosis, antimicrobial therapy, and management of complications: a statement for healthcare professionals from the committee on rheumatic fever, endocarditis, and Kawasaki disease, council on cardiovascular disease in the young, and the councils on clinical cardiology, stroke, and cardiovascular surgery and anesthesia, American heart associates: endorsed by the infectious disease society of America. Circulation 2005:111:394–434.

Chang FY, Peacock JE Jr, Musher DM, et al. *Staphylococcus aureus* bacteremia: recurrence and the impact of antibiotic treatment in prospective multicenter study. Medicine 2003;82:333–339.

Stryhewski ME, Szczech LA, Benjamin DK, et al. Use of vancomycin or first-generation cephalosporins for the treatment of hemodialysis-dependent patients with methicillin-susceptible *Staphylococcus aureus* bacteremia. Clin Infect Dis 2007;44:190–196.

O'Grady N, Alexander M, Burns L, et al. Guidelines for the prevention of intravascular catheter-related infections. Clin Infect Dis 2011;52:e1–21.

Chapter 3c

Candidemia in the Intensive Care Unit

Keith W. Hamilton and Ebbing Lautenbach

Case Presentation

A 62-year-old man with colorectal adenocarcinoma was admitted 4 weeks ago for a right hemicolectomy, complicated by an anastomotic leak. The patient required an exploratory laparotomy 1 week after the initial surgery with peritoneal irrigation and repair of the anastomotic leak. He has been on vancomycin and piperacillin-tazobactam since that time and has remained in the intensive care unit (ICU). Approximately 2 weeks ago, total parenteral nutrition (TPN) via a peripherally inserted central catheter (PICC) was initiated for persistent postoperative ileus. However, approximately 5 days ago the patient developed recurrent fever to 38.7°C. On physical examination, there is no erythema around the PICC, and the abdominal incision is well approximated with no drainage or surrounding erythema. There is a cluster of nontender pustules with erythematous bases on the patient's right thigh. One of four peripheral blood culture vials obtained 3 days ago is growing yeast.

Diagnosis and Initial Management

Yeast in a blood culture should never be considered a contaminant and should be treated promptly with appropriate empiric therapy because delayed treatment has been associated with increased morbidity and mortality. Possible sources should also be investigated. In ICU patients, the most common sources are intravenous catheters and gastrointestinal pathology. In general, *Candida* species are the most common cause of nosocomial invasive fungal infections and are the fourth most common cause of central line-associated blood stream infections overall, representing between 5% and 10%. Risk factors that have been associated with candidemia include: presence of a central venous catheter, TPN, recent gastrointestinal surgery or perforation, receipt of broad-spectrum antibiotics, acute renal failure, hemodialysis, mechanical ventilation, ICU admission, older age, number of red blood cell transfusions, immunosuppression, fungal colonization, and higher severity of illness. Despite advances in treatment and diagnostics, the mortality rates associated with candidemia still remain substantial, with an overall mortality of 30% to over 50% and attributable mortality of 19% to 38%.

Clinical manifestations of candidemia are variable and depend on host immune factors and extent of infection. Symptoms can range from a low-grade fever to sepsis. If skin lesions occur, they often appear as small pustules or nodules with surrounding or overlying erythema, but appearance can be variable, including large, necrotic lesions.

Hematogenous seeding can lead to involvement of heart valves, spleen, liver, central nervous system, joints, and bones. Candidemia can also result in endovascular seeding of the highly vascular choroid plexus in the eye, causing chorioretinitis or endophthalmitis. The possibility of *Candida* chorioretinitis should be evaluated in all patients with candidemia regardless of symptoms because many patients initially lack visual symptoms. Failure to identify this syndrome may result in subsequent loss of vision owing to inappropriate or inadequate duration of treatment, which should be a minimum of 4 to 6 weeks.

Because rapid initiation of antifungal therapy is essential for reducing morbidity and mortality, prompt identification of invasive candidiasis is crucial. Blood cultures have been the standard diagnostic tool, but the sensitivity of standard blood cultures has been questioned. Traditional blood culture methods have a sensitivity of detecting invasive candidiasis of around 50%. However, newer automated culture modalities likely have significantly better performance characteristics. Fungal culture and direct microscopic examination of biopsy or drainage from possible focal sources of infection, including skin lesions and abscesses, provide important additive diagnostic ability. Growth in specialized chromogenic media can expedite the identification of certain *Candida* species.

Desire for more rapid diagnosis has prompted the evaluation of antigen-based assays such as β-D-glucan, which have been used as an adjunct for diagnosis in some invasive fungal infections. The β-D-glucan test detects a cell wall antigen present in most fungi. However, its presence in multiple fungi makes the test less specific for diagnosis of candidemia. The sensitivity ranges from 67% to 100%, and the specificity ranges from 84% to 100%. It can be useful in the appropriate clinical situation, but with careful consideration of its limitations. Consultation with an institution's clinical microbiology department should be initiated to discuss performance characteristics of available diagnostic tools and protocols to optimize chances of isolating *Candida* species.

Traditionally, *C. albicans* has been the most common species involved in nosocomial candidemia, but there has been a progressive shift towards non-albicans *Candida* species, which now outnumber *C. albicans* in many institutions (Table 3.4). Some species such as *C. krusei* are intrinsically resistant to fluconazole and others have variable susceptibility. Physicians must consider the prevalence of individual *Candida* species in addition to their susceptibility profiles in their individual institutions when choosing empiric therapy.

Case Presentation (continued)

The ICU removes the patient's PICC line and obtains surveillance blood cultures. The clinical microbiology laboratory notifies the ICU team that the yeast is likely *C. glabrata* so caspofungin is added to the antimicrobial regimen. A dilated ophthalmologic exam is performed, which reveals no evidence of fungal endophthalmitis or chorioretinitis.

Table 3.4 Common *Candida* Species Associated with Candidemia in the United States						
Species	Percentage of Candida Isolates	Fluconazole Susceptibility	Voriconazole Susceptibility	Posaconazole Susceptibility	Echinocandin Susceptibility	Amphotericin B Susceptibility
C. albicans	45%–58%	S	S	S	S	S
C. glabrata	2%–24%	S-DD to R	S-DD to R	S-DD to R	S	S to I
C. parapsilosis	7%–24%	S	S	S	S to R	S to R
C. tropicalis	11%–16%	S	S	S	S	S
C. krusei	1%–3%	R	S	S	S	S to I
C. lusitaniae	1%–2%	S	S	S	S	S to R

S, susceptible; S-DD, susceptible dose-dependent; I, intermediately susceptible; R, resistant.

Management and Discussion

For infections caused by *C. glabrata*, the preferred empiric agent in many institutions is an echinocandin because of increasing prevalence of *C. glabrata* resistance to fluconazole. Fluconazole should not be used for empiric therapy against *C. glabrata* or other species with high endemic resistance unless the isolate is confirmed to be susceptible. If possible, for all cases of candidemia, metastatic foci should be drained or debrided and gastrointestinal pathology should be repaired. Central venous catheters should be removed as soon as possible, because failure to do so results in higher mortality rates. The duration of therapy for candidemia has not been well studied, but in general, a minimum of 2 weeks of appropriate antifungal therapy from the day of documented clearance of blood cultures and resolution of symptoms is recommended. Longer durations of at least 4 to 6 weeks should be used if there are persistent positive blood cultures, if there has been metastatic seeding, if there are persistent abscesses, if there is focal involvement of deep tissues or organs, or if there is an endovascular focus such as endocarditis. Surgical intervention often plays a critical role in effectively treating these complications.

Especially when clusters of candidemia develop in an institution, infection control personnel should become involved. Some studies have suggested that colonization or infection of patients with *Candida* species could be caused by cross-contamination from healthcare workers. In addition, some outbreaks have also been linked to clonal isolates of various *Candida* species, indicating a common source or horizontal transmission. Regardless of whether clusters are clonal, any increase in candidemia rates in a hospital can be a sign of general lapses in infection control measures. Therefore, infection control procedures including line care, hand hygiene, and universal precautions should be reinforced. Most clusters of candidemia have been halted by institution of these measures. Antifungal prophylaxis has been considered in high-risk patients in order to decrease the rates of nosocomial candidemia, but on the basis of current evidence, there is no data to support this practice in immunocompetent patients, except in certain compelling situations such as necrotizing pancreatitis or gastrointestinal perforation.

Case Conclusion

Blood cultures subsequent to PICC removal remain negative, and the patient has no subsequent fevers. The *C. glabrata* isolate is found to be susceptible to fluconazole so his antifungal regimen is changed to fluconazole, and he is treated for 2 weeks from the first negative blood culture.

Suggested Reading

Blumberg HM, Jarvis WR, Soucie JM, et al. Risk factors for candidal bloodstream infections in surgical intensive care unit patients: the NEMIS prospective multicenter study. The national epidemiology of mycosis survey. Clin Infect Dis 2001;33:177–186.

Chow JK, Golan Y, Ruthazer R, et al. Risk factors for albicans and non-albicans candidemia in the intensive care unit. Crit Care Med 2008;36:1993–1998.

Falagas ME, Roussos N, Vardakas KZ. Relative frequency of albicans and the various non-albicans Candida spp among candidemia isolates from inpatients in various parts of the world: a systematic review. Int J Infect Dis 2010;14:e954–966.

Garey KW, Rege M, Pai MP, et al. Time to initiation of fluconazole therapy impacts mortality in patients with candidemia: a multi-institutional study. Clin Infect Dis 2006;43:25–31.

Hernández-Castro R, Arroyo-Escalante S, Carrillo-Casas EM, et al. Outbreak of Candida parapsilosis in a neonatal intensive care unit: a health care workers source. Eur J Pediatr 2010;169:783–787.

Kuhn DM, Mikherjee PK, Clark TA, et al. Candida parapsilosis characterization in an outbreak setting. Emerg Infect Dis 2004;1074–1081.

Méan M, Marchetti O, Calandra T. Bench-to-bedside review: Candida infections in the intensive care unit. Critical Care 2008;12:204.

Morgan J, Meltzer MI, Plikaytis BD, et al. Excess mortality, hospital stay, and cost due to candidemia: a case-control study using data from population-based candidemia surveillance. Infect Control Hosp Epidemiol 2005;26:540–547.

Montagna MT, Caggiano G, Borghi E, Morace G. The role of the laboratory in the diagnosis of invasive candidiasis. Drugs 2009;69(Suppl 1):59–63.

Ortega M, Marco F, Soriano A, et al. Candida species bloodstream infection: epidemiology and outcome in a single institution from 1991 to 2008. J Hosp Infect 2011;77:157–161.

Pappas PG, Kauffman CA, Andes D, et al. Clinical practice guidelines for the management of candidiasis: 2009 update by the Infectious Diseases Society of America. Clin Infect Dis 2009;48:503–535.

Playford EG, Lipman J, Sorrell TC, et al. Prophylaxis, empirical and preemptive treatment of invasive candidiasis. Curr Opin Crit Care 2010;16:470–474.

Wisplinghoff H, Bischoff T, Tallent SM, et al. Nosocomial bloodstream infections in US hospitals: analysis of 24,179 cases from a prospective nationwide surveillance study. Clin Infect Dis 2004;39:309–317.

Chapter 3d

Central Line Tunnel Infections

Michael J. Satlin and David P. Calfee

Case Presentation

A 65-year old man with end-stage renal disease from hypertension and diabetes mellitus who receives hemodialysis through a right internal jugular, tunneled catheter presents to his outpatient dialysis unit with 2 days of fever and chills. He has no symptoms referable to the respiratory, urinary, or gastrointestinal tracts and last received hemodialysis 2 days prior. The catheter was placed 2 months ago and has been functioning properly. An arteriovenous fistula was created one month ago in his left wrist and is awaiting maturation before use. His diabetes and hypertension are well controlled on oral agents and he has no medication allergies.

On initial examination, he is febrile (38.4°C) but all other vital signs are normal. He has erythema and tenderness along the entire subcutaneous portion of the tunneled catheter without significant induration or fluctuance. No purulence is visible at the catheter exit site. The remainder of his physical examination is normal.

Diagnosis

The differential diagnosis of fever and chills in a patient with diabetes undergoing hemodialysis is broad, including vascular access-related infection, upper respiratory tract infection, pneumonia, urinary tract infection, and diabetic foot infection. However, in this patient, the lack of other symptoms coupled with the physical exam finding of an erythematous and tender catheter tunnel tract strongly suggest a catheter-related infection. A tunnel infection is distinguished from a catheter exit site infection in that the tenderness, erythema, and induration are more than 2 cm from the catheter exit site, as in this case. Tunnel infections can exist with or without accompanying bloodstream infection. If significant induration or fluctuance is noted on exam, an ultrasound should be considered to assess for a fluid collection that may require drainage.

Two sets of blood cultures are indicated in this case to determine whether the patient is simultaneously bacteremic and to guide antimicrobial therapy. Ideally, at least one set should be obtained from a peripheral vein, preferably one that will not be used for a dialysis fistula or graft (because venipuncture can injure the vein). In cases without overt signs of tunnel or exit site infection but where catheter-related bloodstream infection (CRBSI) is suspected, simultaneous collection of blood cultures from the catheter and a peripheral vein may be helpful to determine whether the catheter is the source of the infection. The presence of microbial growth in the catheter culture at least 2 hours before growth in the peripheral culture, known as *differential time to positivity*, provides strong evidence for CRBSI. When a peripheral blood sample cannot be obtained, two sets of cultures may be drawn from the dialysis catheter or tubing. If an exudate is apparent at the catheter exit site, a sample of the exudate should be obtained for gram stain and culture. Whenever possible, all cultures should be obtained before initiating empiric antimicrobial therapy.

It is important to note that signs of a tunnel infection in neutropenic oncology patients may be more subtle, presenting with minimal erythema, tenderness, or fluctuance. Therefore, clinicians caring for a patient with a tunneled catheter who presents with fever and neutropenia should perform a careful examination of the catheter to detect subtle signs of tunnel infection. In all patients with suspected CRBSI, a careful history and physical examination, and additional testing when appropriate, should be performed to rule out metastatic complications, such as osteomyelitis, endocarditis, septic arthritis, and epidural abscess. Metastatic complications are particularly common in patients with *Staphylococcus aureus* CRBSI.

Case Presentation (continued)

After collecting two sets of blood cultures, one from a peripheral vein and one from the catheter, intravenous vancomycin (20 mg/kg) and gentamicin (1 mg/kg) are infused through the catheter. The tunneled catheter is removed and a temporary, untunneled dialysis catheter is placed by interventional radiology. The patient is admitted to the hospital for observation and undergoes dialysis the next day through the new catheter. Two new sets of blood cultures are drawn during dialysis. He is afebrile after removal of the tunneled catheter and is discharged after dialysis. Later that day, both sets of initial blood cultures are reported as positive for microbial growth. The initial gram stain demonstrates gram-positive cocci in clusters, which are subsequently identified as oxacillin-resistant, vancomycin-susceptible *Staphylococcus epidermidis*. At each subsequent dialysis session during the next 10 days, he is given 500 mg of intravenous vancomycin. His repeat blood cultures are negative, the inflammation along the prior tunnel tract resolves, and a new, tunneled dialysis catheter is placed.

Management and Discussion

The antimicrobial therapy administered in this case was appropriate. Although coagulase-negative *Staphylococcus* and *Staphylococcus aureus* are the most common causes of CRBSI in hemodialysis patients with tunneled catheters, gram-negative rods and enterococci are also important causes of these infections. The microbial etiologies of tunnel infections have not been well described, although staphylococci are thought to be most common. Given the spectrum of potential bacterial pathogens, empiric antimicrobial therapy for tunneled dialysis catheter infections should provide gram-positive and gram-negative coverage. In general, agents with pharmacokinetic characteristics that permit dosing in conjunction with dialysis sessions are preferred to avoid placement of an additional intravenous catheter. Vancomycin is appropriate empiric therapy for gram-positive coverage given the high prevalence of oxacillin resistance among coagulase-negative *Staphylococcus* and *S. aureus*. Ceftazidime or gentamicin is appropriate for empiric gram-negative coverage in the absence of information that suggests a high likelihood of a gram-negative organism resistant to one of these agents (e.g., prior infection with cephalosporin-resistant *Escherichia coli*). The pharmacokinetics of these agents allow for dosing after dialysis sessions (Table 3.5). Antimicrobial therapy should be adjusted as appropriate as blood culture results become available. In particular, patients with CRBSI caused by methicillin-susceptible *S. aureus* (MSSA) who receive empiric treatment with vancomycin should be switched to an antistaphylococcal β-lactam because of greater rates of treatment failure with vancomycin compared to antistaphylococcal β-lactams. In the Infectious Diseases Society of America (IDSA) guidelines, cefazolin is the β-lactam recommended for the treatment of dialysis catheter-related MSSA bloodstream infection based on data supporting its effectiveness when administered only after dialysis sessions (see Table 3.5).

In patients undergoing hemodialysis through a tunneled catheter, CRBSI poses a unique challenge because a functional catheter is required for ongoing

77

Table 3.5 Antimicrobial Agents that can be Administered in Conjunction with Hemodialysis sessions and Recommended Adult Dosing for Hemodialysis Catheter-related Bloodstream Infections

Antimicrobial Agent	Dosing
Vancomycin	15–20 mg/kg loading dose,[a] followed by:
	500 mg at the end of each subsequent dialysis session OR
	Obtain serum vancomycin concentration prior to dialysis and administer 500–1,000 mg at the end of dialysis only if the level is below or within the desired trough range[b]
Cefazolin	20 mg/kg after each dialysis session[c]
Ceftazidime	1 g after each dialysis session
Gentamicin	1–2 mg/kg initial dose (not to exceed 100 mg)[c], followed by:
	1–2 mg/kg after each dialysis session[d] OR
	Obtain a serum gentamicin concentration prior to dialysis and dose 1–2 mg/kg after dialysis if the level is <2 µg/ml

CRBSI, catheter elated bloodstream infections.

[a]Dosing based on actual body weight.

[b]Consider monitoring serum vancomycin concentrations in severe cases of CRBSI or cases complicated by endocarditis or osteomyelitis.

[c]Dosing based on ideal or adjusted body weight.

[d]Consider monitoring serum gentamicin concentrations in patients receiving longer courses of gentamicin therapy (e.g., >5 days).

dialysis. All such patients should receive intravenous antimicrobial therapy, but there are a number of options for management of the infected catheter: (1) prompt catheter removal with delayed placement of a new tunneled catheter, (2) exchange of the infected catheter with a new one over a guidewire, and (3) attempted salvage of the catheter by administering antimicrobial lock therapy at each dialysis session in addition to systemic therapy. Antimicrobial lock therapy consists of instilling a high concentration of an antimicrobial to which the causative microbe is susceptible into the catheter lumen, with the goal of achieving local antimicrobial concentrations that are high enough to kill microbes growing within the catheter biofilm. If the catheter is compatible with ethanol, some might consider an ethanol lock instead of an antibiotic lock solution, although this is not included in current IDSA guidelines. Administration of intravenous antimicrobials alone, without catheter removal, exchange, or antimicrobial lock therapy is not recommended because of high rates of treatment failure and infection recurrence with this strategy. In the presence of a catheter tunnel infection, such as in this case, the catheter should be removed and a temporary dialysis catheter should be placed (option 1). A new, tunneled hemodialysis catheter can be placed once blood cultures with negative results are obtained. Other scenarios where catheter removal is preferred are cases of severe sepsis or CRBSI due to *S. aureus*, *Pseudomonas* or *Candida* species.

Although no randomized controlled trials exist to guide the duration of antimicrobial therapy for a hemodialysis catheter tunnel infection, IDSA guidelines recommend 7 to 10 days of therapy after catheter removal for a tunnel infection without concomitant bacteremia or candidemia. In a case such as this one with concomitant bacteremia, the optimal treatment duration is dependent on the pathogen, duration of fever and bacteremia, and the presence of metastatic disease or suppurative thrombophlebitis. Given that this patient was infected with coagulase-negative *Staphylococcus*, promptly defervesced, cleared his blood cultures, and had no complications, a short course of therapy (7–10 days) was reasonable.

The incidence of CRBSI in hemodialysis patients is lower with the use of tunneled, cuffed hemodialysis catheters, compared with untunneled catheters. However, tunneled catheters still carry a greater risk of infection than arteriovenous fistulas and grafts. Thus, permanent surgical arteriovenous access should be pursued and utilized for patients undergoing chronic hemodialysis whenever possible. As with all central venous catheters, proper aseptic technique should be followed while inserting and accessing the catheter to decrease the risk of infection.

Case Conclusion

The patient remained afebrile and asymptomatic throughout and after completion of his antimicrobial course. One month later, it is determined that his arteriovenous fistula is sufficiently mature for use and his tunneled catheter is removed.

Suggested Reading

Allon M. Dialysis catheter-related bacteremia: treatment and prophylaxis. Am J Kidney Dis 2004;44(5):779–791.

Maki DG, Kluger DM, Crnich CJ. The risk of bloodstream infection in adults with different intravascular devices: a systematic review of 200 published prospective studies. Mayo Clin Proc 2006;81(9):1159–1171.

Mermel LA, Allon M, Bouza E, et al. Clinical practice guidelines for the diagnosis and management of intravascular catheter-related infection: 2009 update by the Infectious Diseases Society of America. Clin Infect Dis 2009;49(1):1–45.

Saad TF. Bacteremia associated with tunneled, cuffed hemodialysis catheters. Am J Kidney Dis 1999;34(6):1114–1124.

Sullivan R, Samuel V, Le C, et al. Hemodialysis vascular catheter-related bacteremia. Am J Med Sci 2007;334(6):458–465.

Chapter 3e

Intracardiac Device Infections

Meghan Brennan and Christopher J. Crnich

Case Presentation

A 60 year-old diabetic woman with ischemic cardiomyopathy underwent left ventricular assist device (LVAD) implantation as a bridge to cardiac transplant. A permanent pacemaker (PPM) and intracardiac defibrillator (ICD) were placed at the same time. The patient did well postoperatively, and she was discharged from the hospital within 1 week. Once home, however, she developed pain and swelling over the pacemaker generator pocket as well as chills and anorexia. She called her physician requesting urgent evaluation. In the cardiac transplantation clinic, the patient appeared acutely ill and was febrile to 38.2°C. Her pacemaker pocket site was warm and erythematous with fluctuance around the pacemaker generator on palpation. The LVAD drive-line site did not appear to be inflamed and there was no tenderness over the LVAD pump site.

Differential Diagnosis and Initial Management

Surgical site infections following PPM/ICD implantation are estimated to occur at a rate of 5 per 1,000 device-years.[1] Clinically, they may manifest either as: (1) localized infection of the pacemaker generator pocket, (2) right-sided endocarditis because of infection of transvenous endocardial pacing leads, (3) pericarditis or mediastinitis because of infection of epicardial pacing leads, or (4) some combination thereof. Pacemaker generator pocket infections most commonly arise as a result of device contamination at the time of insertion. In these cases, the onset of infection is typically within 6 months of implantation although later infection may develop following battery replacement.[2] Infections involving pacing leads generally manifest later and may occur either as a result of: (1) lead contamination at the time of implantation, (2) migration of microorganisms from an infected pacemaker generator pocket, or (3) hematogenous seeding as a result of bacteremia originating from another site of infection (e.g., pneumonia).[2]

Staphylococcus aureus or coagulase-negative staphylococci (CoNS) are recovered in 80% to 90% of microbiologically confirmed episodes of PPM/ICD infection[2] although *Propionobacterium acnes* has been increasingly recognized as a cause of infection.[3] Recovery of gram-negative bacteria from patients with a

PPM/ICD infection is uncommon and almost always occurs in the setting of an early post-implantation wound infection. Late infections secondary to hematogenous seeding of the implant are almost always caused by gram-positive bacteria as gram-negative bacteria seldom cause infection by this route.[4]

Patients with pacemaker generator pocket infections usually present with localized warmth, swelling, redness, and tenderness involving the skin over the device, as was described in this case. Systemic signs and symptoms are variably present. Infection of pacing leads may be associated with fulminant septicemia when caused by aggressive organisms like *S. aureus* but may follow a more indolent pattern when caused by CoNS or *P. acnes*. In either case, signs and symptoms of right-sided endocarditis are often present, including fever and chills (in >80% of cases), septic pulmonary emboli (20% to 45%), and tricuspid regurgitation (25%).[2]

Initial management of suspected PPM/ICD infection involves a prompt diagnostic evaluation followed by early initiation of empiric antimicrobial therapy (see Fig. 3.4). Blood cultures should be obtained to rule out the presence of bacteremia, and fluid aspirated percutaneously from around the pacer generator should be cultured in order to guide antimicrobial therapy. If blood cultures are positive, transesophageal echocardiography should be performed to establish the extent of endocardial involvement (e.g., ring abscess, valvular incompetence) and need for more aggressive surgical management. Chest imaging with either CT or MR may be required to evaluate for pericarditis or mediastinitis in patients with suspected infection of epicardial pacing leads, especially if signs and symptoms of infection do not improve with the administration of appropriate

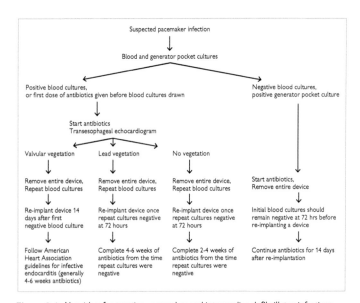

Figure 3.4 Algorithm for treating pacemaker and intracardiac defibrillator infections. (American Heart Association guidelines for infective endocarditis can be found at http://circ. ahajournals.org/cgi/content/full/111/23/e394)

antimicrobial therapy. Empiric antimicrobial therapy targeting gram-positive bacteria, including methicillin-resistant *Staphylococcus aureus* (MRSA), should be initiated after cultures have been obtained. Empiric coverage for nosocomial gram-negative bacteria (i.e., *Pseudomonas*) should be considered for infections that develop in the early post-implantation period (<2 months following implantation).

In the current case, the patient's malaise and fever raised suspicion for concurrent bacteremia, and the overall picture was further complicated by the presence of an LVAD. Infection following LVAD placement is common—0.5 events per patient-year—and may involve any component of the device.[5]

Infection of the skin at the drive line exit site is the most commonly encountered infectious complication of LVADs. Patients with LVAD drive line infections typically present with erythema and purulence at the exit site although these findings can also be present in patients with severe local irritation even in the absence of infection. Differentiating the two requires close monitoring for progressive erythema and drainage, as well as the presence of accompanying signs and symptoms of systemic infection. Infections of the LVAD pump pocket may arise either as a result of device contamination at the time of implantation or as a result of direct extension from an infected drive line. Patients often have local signs of infection (e.g., pain and swelling) and may present with varying degrees of systemic symptoms, depending on the infecting organism. Imaging with either ultrasound or CT, and aspiration of periimplant fluid collections are critical from a diagnostic and therapeutic standpoint in these situations. The most feared infectious complication of LVAD use is involvement of the endovascular components. The endovascular LVAD components may become infected as a result of contamination at the time of implantation but are particularly prone to hematogenous seeding as a result of the large surface area in direct contact with blood and the nonlaminar flow created by the complicated surface structure of the device.[5]

Staphylococci are the predominant causes of LVAD infections although a significant proportion of microbiologically confirmed cases may be caused by enterococci, *Pseudomonas* spp., *enterobacteriaceae, and Candida* spp.[5] Management of patients with a suspected LVAD infection requires a prompt evaluation with blood cultures, culture of fluid discharge from the drive line exit site and sampling of fluid from the pump pocket, if clinically indicated. Once cultures have been obtained, broad-spectrum empiric antimicrobial therapy that includes coverage for gram-positive (MRSA and enterococci), gram-negative (*Pseudomonas*), and *Candida* coverage should be initiated. A typical empiric antimicrobial regimen at our institution includes vancomycin (dosed for a target trough of 15–20 μg/ml) combined with an anti-pseudomonal β-lactam and ciprofloxacin. Fluconazole or an echinocandin may be added to this regimen in patients with a documented history of yeast infections or recent intensive antibiotic exposure (e.g., those patients being treated for a prior LVAD infection).

Case Presentation (continued)

The patient was diagnosed with a pacemaker pocket infection on the basis of her clinical presentation. However, an endovascular infection involving her pacer leads and/or LVAD components was also suspected. Blood cultures were obtained and a percutaneous aspirate of fluid from the pacemaker generator pocket was performed in the clinic. The patient received a stat dose of intravenous vancomycin after cultures were collected. She was admitted to the hospital where vancomycin was continued and intravenous cefepime and oral ciprofloxacin were added to her empiric regimen. The microbiology laboratory contacted the admitting team within 12 hours to report that blood cultures were growing gram-positive cocci in clusters, which were subsequently confirmed to be MRSA. Culture of the pacemaker pocket also grew MRSA. A transesophageal echocardiogram revealed no vegetations. Although the LVAD remained free of overt signs of infection, it was presumed to be infected prompting escalation of her transplant status. She was subsequently treated with "suppressive" vancomycin until heart transplantation 6 months later, during which she underwent simultaneous explantation of the pacemaker, ICD, and LVAD. Cultures of the explanted LVAD pump and pacemaker generator both grew MRSA. The patient was treated for three additional weeks of vancomycin to target residual infection in the device beds.

Management and Discussion

Medical therapy alone will rarely cure a PPM/ICD or LVAD infection. The complex biofilm that develops on implanted devices such as PPM/ICDs and LVADs inhibits the penetration and activity of most systemic antibiotics. A combined medical and surgical approach that involves partial or complete removal of the device is necessary to achieve definitive cure in most situations.[6] The presence of a mature biofilm explains why, even after 6 months of appropriate antibiotic therapy, live organisms were able to be cultured from the LVAD and pacemaker generator in the current case.

When confronted with an isolated pacemaker infection, the entire device should be removed. Even if the infection is thought to be isolated to the generator pocket, limited debridement and prolonged antibiotic use is associated with unacceptably high relapse rates.[7] When the infection involves epicardial leads, device removal is of paramount importance. Medical management alone is associated with a mortality rate of 41%, whereas a combined approach with complete removal of the device yields 18% mortality.

While removing pacing leads clearly reduces the risk for relapsed infection, the procedure is not without risk. A fibrinous sheath may develop around leads that have been implanted for an extended period of time, and traction alone can fail to dislodge such leads. In these instances, open-heart surgery may be required. However, a new excimer laser sheath has been shown to be particularly effective in removing leads while using a minimally invasive approach. Another potential complication is that of septic emboli from leads encumbered with large vegetations. The concern is that extracting the leads through a narrow insertion path will dislodge the vegetation when it is still in the cardiac chamber, leading to pulmonary embolization. While this may occur, the vast majority of patients undergoing removal in the setting of even large vegetations generally remain asymptomatic and tolerate the procedure well. Still, some authorities suggest surgical extraction if the leads are compromised by vegetations larger than 10 mm in size.[7] Surgical management should be coupled with prompt empiric antibiotics that can ultimately be narrowed based on culture results. Duration of therapy is dependent on the extent of infection.

In the case of LVAD infection, management is complicated by the need to maintain continuous cardiovascular support, making immediate device removal an impossibility in most cases. Simple drive line exit site infections can often be managed with local wound care and a defined course of antibiotics—typically about 14 days—until healing has occurred, although recurrence in these situations remains common. More complicated infections almost always require indefinite suppressive antibiotic therapy until the LVAD can be explanted, typically at the time of transplantation.[5] The increasing use of LVADs in patients who will never become candidates for transplantation—generally referred to as "destination therapy" —represents a particularly challenging clinical situation. Indefinite parenteral therapy is usually not an option, but discontinuation of systemic therapy in these cases is associated with a high rate of relapse and extension of infection. Stepdown to oral suppressive therapy following an intensive course of parenteral therapy is theoretically possible but the experience and outcomes associated with this approach are limited. The involvement of an infectious disease specialist with experience in treating implant-associated infections can be particularly helpful in identifying the factors (Table 3.6) that can influence the likelihood of success with different management options.

Given the disastrous complications associated with intracardiac device infections, prevention is particularly important. Maintaining surgical asepsis during insertion has been shown to reduce the risk of PPM/ICD infection and prophylactic administration of anti-staphylococcal antibiotics is of proven benefit. Perioperative antibiotic regimens for LVAD implantation should provide

Table 3.6 General Considerations Influencing Treatment Strategies for LVAD Infections

Site of Infection

Superficial infections around the drive line exit site may be cured with a 14-day course of antibiotics, but deeper sites usually benefit from prolonged therapy.

Pathogen

S. aureus and Pseudomonas are more virulent organisms and more likely to cause symptomatic breakthrough infections when treated with oral antibiotics. As such, they are more likely to require prolonged parenteral therapy.

Antimicrobial Susceptibilities

If a Pseudomonal strain is fluoroquinolone susceptible, ciprofloxacin may offer an excellent oral stepdown option because of its high bioavailability.

Patient

Whether the LVAD is intended as a bridge to transplantation or not ("destination LVAD") impacts if and when to transfer to oral suppressive therapy. When the patient is listed for transplantation, extending parenteral therapy is reasonable given that cure (with device removal at the time of transplantation and aggressive antimicrobials) is feasible. When the patient is not listed for transplantation, the goal of therapy shifts from cure to suppression. At this point, transitioning to an oral regimen is a higher priority.

coverage for skin organisms (staphylococci and streptococci), with some authorities routinely recommending broader, additional coverage for gram-negative bacteria and *Candida*.[8] Preoperative MRSA screening and decontamination may reduce risk further but have not been specifically studied in this patient population.

Case Conclusion

The patient did very well after transplantation. Antibiotics were stopped after 3 weeks, and there have been no signs of recurrent infection.

References

Johansen JB, Jorgensen OD, Moller M Arnsbo P, Mortensen PT, Nielsen JC. Infection after pacemaker implantation: infection rates and risk factors associated with infection in a population-based cohort study of 46299 consecutive patients. Eur Heart J 2011;32:991–998.

Crnich CJ, Safdar N, Maki DM. Infections associated with implanted medical devices. In: Finch RG, Greenwood D, Norrby SR, Whitle RJ, eds. Antibiotics and chemotherapy: anti-infective agents and their uses in therapy, 8th ed. New York: Churchill Livingston, 2003:575–618.

Zedtwitz-Liebenstein K, Gabriel H, Graninger W. Pacemaker endocarditis due to Propionibacterium acnes. Infection 2003;31(3):184–185.

Uslan, DZ, Sohail MR, Friedman PA, Heyes DL, Wilson WR, Steckelberg JM, et al. Frequency of permanent pacemaker or implantable cardioverter-defibrillator infection in patients with gram-negative bacteremia. Clin Infect Dis 2006;43(6):731–736.

Gordon RJ, Quagliarello B, Lowy FD. Ventricular assist device related infections. Lancet Infect Dis 2006;6:426–437.

Hall-Stoodley L, Costerton JW, Stoodley P. Bacterial biofilms: from the natural environment to infectious disease. Nat Rev Microbiol 2004;2(2):95–108.

Sohail MR, Sultan OW, Raza SS. Contemporary management of cardiovascular implantable electronic device infections. Expert Rev Anti Infect Ther 2010;8(7):831–839.

Rose EA, Gelijns AC, Moskowitz AJ, Heitjan DF, Stevenson LW, Dembitsky W, et al. Long-term use of a left ventricular assist device for end-stage heart failure. NEJM 2001;(20):1435–1443.

Chapter 3f

Arteriovenous Fistula and Graft Infections

Natasha Bagdasarian, Michael Heung, and Preeti N. Malani

Initial Case Presentation

A 51 year old man with end-stage renal disease (ESRD) on maintenance hemo-dialysis presented to his dialysis unit with fevers and pain at the site of his dialy-sis access, a right upper extremity arteriovenous graft (AVG). He had no other localizing symptoms. His comorbidities included hypertension, diabetes mel-litus, and peripheral vascular disease. Vascular access history was notable for multiple previous failed surgical accesses in his left upper extremity, attributed to a central venous stenosis that was not amenable to intervention.

On physical exam, temperature was 101.2°F and blood pressure 140/95, which was consistent with baseline. His right upper extremity AVG site was slightly warm and tender, but without significant erythema or fluctuance. His AVG was accessed for dialysis initiation without difficulty, and two sets of blood cultures were obtained. He was also started empirically on vancomycin, 1.5 grams administered during the final hour of his dialysis session. Within 12 hours, blood cultures demonstrated growth of methicillin-resistant *Staphylococcus aureus* (MRSA). The minimum inhibitory concentration (MIC) for vancomycin was 2 μg/ml. Vancomycin therapy was continued with a plan for 6 weeks of therapy. On therapy, the patient reported some improvement in his right arm pain, and surveillance blood cultures 1 and 2 weeks later were negative.

Differential Diagnosis and Initial Management

Although gram-negative and fungal infections do occur, gram-positive cocci are responsible for the vast majority of hemodialysis-related (HD) infections. Coagulase-negative *Staphylococcus* (CONS) is responsible for most catheter-related bloodstream infections (CRBSI), while *S. aureus* is more common with arteriovenous fistula (AVF) or graft (AVG) infections. *S. aureus* is more often associated with treatment failure and infectious complications of CRBSI.

Although there are specific criteria for the diagnosis of a CRBSI, the diagno-sis is often presumed when a symptomatic patient with an indwelling hemodi-alysis catheter has positive catheter-drawn and/or peripheral blood culture and no other identifiable source of infection. Infections of an AVF or AVG are much less common, and may be more difficult to diagnose. The access site may demonstrate local erythema, pain, and warmth; however, AV access infections may be occult. When there is a high clinical suspicion for access associated infection (e.g., persistent bacteremia without another obvious source or relapsed bacteremia), imaging with ultrasound and/or indium scanning may be helpful, although the sensitivity and specificity of this approach is not well established.

Once infection is suspected or confirmed, appropriate antimicrobial selection and administration is essential. Antimicrobial dosing is particularly problematic among ESRD patients. For example, vancomycin kinetics can be affected by the type of dialysis filter, duration of and intervals between sessions, body weight, and residual renal function. Whereas low levels can be associated with treatment failures and the development of resistance, high levels can result in toxicity. Duration of treatment depends on the clinical scenario, including the organism isolated, presence of infectious complications, and decision regarding access removal versus salvage. If there is no evidence to suggest complicated infection and/or endocarditis, the duration of therapy generally consists of 2 to 4 weeks of parenteral treatment. Many factors can impact treatment duration, especially in the setting of relapsed or recurrent infection.

Case Presentation (continued)

Four months later, the patient presented again with fever and discomfort at the AVG site. Empiric therapy with vancomycin was initiated. Blood culture confirmed recurrent MRSA bacteremia (vancomycin MIC 4 µg/ml). Despite the antimicrobial therapy, the patient continued to experience intermittent low-grade fevers. Follow-up cultures 1 week after initial presentation demonstrated persistent bacteremia. The patient was admitted for surgical and infectious disease evaluation. Antimicrobials were switched from vancomycin to daptomycin. Ultrasound of his AVG site showed tissue inflammation but no fluid pockets. Transesophageal echocardiogram was negative for endocarditis. After extensive discussion, the patient's infected AVG was surgically removed. Blood cultures demonstrated subsequent clearing. He had a tunneled dialysis catheter placed and was discharged to complete an additional 4 weeks of daptomycin therapy. He was later reassessed for a new surgical access and a femoral AVG was recommended due to lack of remaining upper extremity options. The patient declined this option and thus remained catheter-dependent.

Management and Discussion

More than 380,000 patients are currently receiving maintenance dialysis in the United States. Despite significant advances in dialysis care and overall survival, infections related to dialysis access remain the "Achilles heel" of ESRD management. The type of access is perhaps the most important determinant of infection risk. Table 3.7 provides an overview of the different vascular access options available for HD patients, including risk of infection. The preferred access is generally AVF because of highest long-term patency rates and lowest infection

Table 3.7 Vascular Access for Hemodialysis

Access Type		Characteristics	
Arteriovenous fistula (AVF): Surgically created connection between native artery and vein	Access of choice for chronic HD	Highest long-term patency rate Associated with lowest infection rates compared to other access options	High primary failure rate Long maturation period (~2–3 months)
Arteriovenous graft (AVG): Exogenous tube placed subcutaneously to connect artery and vein	Second choice access for chronic HD	Faster maturation (3–4 weeks post placement) Higher early patency rates than AVF	Higher infectious risk than AVF Lower long-term patency rate than AVF
Tunneled dialysis catheter: Central venous catheter with subcutaneous tract ("tunnel") between vascular insertion and exit site	For patients who do not have a mature AVF or AVG at time of HD initiation	Can be used immediately	Higher infection risk than AVF or AVG Access related-complications (clotting, etc.)
Acute (non-tunneled) dialysis catheter: Central venous catheter	Reserved for in-hospital acute HD; temporary access	Easy to place (no need for fluoroscopy) Can be used immediately	Highest infection risk

ESRD, end stage renal disease; HD, hemodialysis.

risk, whereas the next best option is generally an AVG. Intravascular catheters are associated with the highest incidence of complications, including CRBSI.

After first initiating antimicrobial therapy for CRBSI, the dialysis catheter should be removed in the setting of sepsis, tunnel infection, hematogenous spread of infection, prolonged bacteremia, or for infections associated with difficult-to-eradicate organisms including S. aureus, Pseudomonas aeruginosa, fungi, and mycobacteria. Infections of an AVF can usually be treated with long courses of antimicrobials alone, whereas AVG infections may require surgical resection in addition to antimicrobial therapy.

Access removal is complicated by a variety of issues unique to dialysis-dependent patients. Dialysis access essentially functions as a "life-line." Therefore, the risk of losing vascular access will often result in reluctance to opt for early removal. The possibility of an access-free interval is limited by the need for regular and routine dialysis. Last, because of prior access-related interventions and/or vascular disease (which is prevalent in ESRD patients), there may be limited sites for access replacement.

If access salvage is attempted, long courses of antimicrobial therapy are sometimes used. In this setting, the notion of "MIC creep" (decreased susceptibility to vancomycin that develops while on therapy) is of particular significance. Maintenance dialysis therapy is one of the most significant risk factors for infections with vancomycin-intermediate and even vancomycin-resistant S. aureus strains. Acquisition of these highly resistant strains is also linked to receipt of multiple, extended courses of vancomycin, particularly when trough levels are consistently subtherapeutic. Current treatment guidelines now recommend higher trough targets (15–20 mcg/ml) when treating MRSA bacteremia.

While a long-term tunneled dialysis catheter is not optimal for several reasons including the higher risk of infection, antimicrobial locks are a promising strategy to reduce the risk of recurrent CRBSI among catheter-dependent patients. The most recent CRBSI prevention guidelines provide a stronger recommendation for antimicrobial lock use among patients who develop recurrent infection in spite of optimal adherence to aseptic technique. This technique involves filling the catheter lumen with a lock solution and allowing it to remain in place when the catheter is not being used. Lock solutions include antibiotics (most notably vancomycin) as well as other agents (e.g., ethanol and recombinant tissue plasminogen activator). Recently, a novel lock solution containing sodium citrate, methylene blue, methylparaben, and propylparaben (C-MB-P), has shown promise in hemodialysis patients. Studies to better define the best agents and most appropriate indications for use are ongoing.

Case Conclusion

After recovering from the infection, the patient was reassessed for a new surgical access and a femoral AVG was recommended due to lack of remaining upper extremity options. However, the patient declined this option and thus remained catheter-dependent.

Suggested Reading

Akoh JA. Vascular access infections: epidemiology, diagnosis, and management. Curr Infect Dis Rep 2011;13:324–332.

Fitzgibbons LN, Puls DL, Mackay K, Forrest GN. Management of gram-positive coccal bacteremia and hemodialysis. Am J Kidney Dis 2011;57:624–640.

Maki DG, Ash SR, Winger RK, Lavin P. A novel antimicrobial and antithrombotic lock solution for hemodialysis catheters: a multi-center, controlled, randomized trial. Crit Care Med 2011;39:613–620.

Patel PR, Kallen AJ, Arduino MJ. Epidemiology, surveillance, and prevention of bloodstream infections in hemodialysis patients. Am J Kidney Dis 2010;56:566–577.

Schild AF, Perez E, Gillaspie E, Seaver C, Livingstone J, Thibonnier A. Arteriovenous fistulae vs. arteriovenous grafts: a retrospective review of 1,700 consecutive vascular access cases. J Vasc Access. 2008;9:231–235.

Chapter 4a

Necrotizing Fasciitis after Surgery

Rebekah Moehring and Stephen G. Weber

Initial Case Presentation

A 44-year-old man presents to the emergency department with complaint of sudden onset of abdominal pain and nausea. He is febrile (38.5°C) and pain is localized to the right upper quadrant. Sonogram reveals an inflamed gallbladder. Labs collected in the ER reveal a severe leukocytosis. He is taken to the operating room where an urgent open cholecystectomy is performed, revealing a nonperforated gallbladder. A preoperative antibiotic, cefazolin, was administered within 1 hour prior to incision. After a brief stay in the recovery room, he is transferred to the general surgery inpatient unit. He rests comfortably overnight receiving analgesia and intravenous antibiotics.

By the next morning, the patient is complaining of fever (38.9°C) and tenderness at the surgical site. The wound appears to be intact and on morning rounds the surgeon is generally satisfied with the patient's progress. However, 3 hours later, his temperature is 39.4°C and he has rigors. The primary nurse alerts the surgeon that there is an area of erythema extending from the surgical wound inferiorly that was not present when her shift began 3 hours earlier. The patient's blood pressure has dropped to 90/55 mmHg, and his pulse increased to 114 beats per minute.

Differential Diagnosis and Initial Management

Surgical site infection (SSI) is one of the most common types of healthcare associated infections encountered in clinical practice, occurring in 2% to 5% of patients undergoing inpatient surgery in the United States.[1] The severity of SSI can range from simple, superficial cellulitis or stitch abscess to life-threatening, invasive infections involving the deep organ space.[2] Several features of this case suggest that more severe infection may be at play. Although fever within 48 hours after abdominal surgery can be anticipated even in the absence of infection,[2] the degree of the temperature elevation, along with the accompanying rigors and leukocytosis require a higher level of concern. The nurse's observation of erythema *developing and spreading rapidly* at the surgical site as well as instability of the patient's vital signs raises an alarm for necrotizing fasciitis.

Necrotizing fasciitis (NF) is the most feared of skin and soft tissue infections and is frequently lethal, with mortality estimates ranging 30% to 67%.[3] Categorical typing of NF has been proposed based on the causative organism(s) and clinical presentation.[3,4] Most (70%–80%) of NF cases are type I. Type I NF is characterized by polymicrobial infection that is progressive over a period of days and often associated with underlying immunocompromised state or abdominal pathology, including recent abdominal surgery.[3,5] Type II NF is generally monomicrobial and includes the most severe and highly fatal cases associated with toxin-producing strains of gram-positive bacteria, particularly group A streptococci (GAS). Aggressive, contiguous spread of soft tissue necrosis accompanied by overwhelming sepsis specifically characterizes GAS NF. Approximately half of GAS NF cases are associated with streptococcal toxic shock syndrome, which increases mortality rates to 67%.[3]

Symptoms of NF can occur so rapidly that it seems spontaneous, and definitive diagnosis may be elusive. An attentive clinician with a high index of suspicion,

Table 4.1 Four Essential Keys to the Management of Necrotizing Fasciitis	
Early Identification	• Clinical judgment is the most important element of diagnosis.
	• Classic Clinical Findings (in order of early to late findings):
	• Systemic signs of sepsis ± shock
	• Rapid progression
	• Pain out of proportion to physical exam findings
	• Erythema and tense edema of the involved skin, sometimes described as "wooden"
	• Purplish or dark-colored bullae and blisters
	• Crepitus (10%) and subcutaneous gas
	• Central anesthesia of involved skin
	• CT or MRI confirmation of diagnosis is NOT recommended if clinical suspicion is high.
	• Delay in operative management is associated with higher mortality.
	• Operative finding of tissue necrosis confirms the diagnosis.
Surgical Source Control	• **Urgent operative debridement** of devitalized tissues is required.
	• Repeat exploration and debridement within 24–48 hours.
	• May require multiple daily surgeries until advancing necrosis is halted.
	• Management with antibiotics alone approaches 100% mortality
Antibiotics	• Immediate initiation of **empiric broad coverage** of aerobic gram-positive, aerobic gram-negative, and anaerobic pathogens
	• Addition of **clindamycin** for protein synthesis inhibition—especially if clostridium or group A streptococcus is suspected
	• Target therapy based on operative and blood cultures.
Supportive Care	• Aggressive fluid resuscitation for signs of shock
	• ICU management is often required.
	• Vasopressors may be required in cases of Streptococcal or Staphylococcal toxic shock syndrome.

performing serial physical exams, is often essential to timely diagnosis. Table 4.1 lists the classic clinical findings of NF: systemic sepsis, rapidly progressive skin erythema, and edema, disproportionate pain, bullae or blisters, subcutaneous air and crepitus. However, these exam findings are insensitive (present in just 10%–40% of cases), may occur alone or together, and are often relatively late manifestations of serious infection.[3,6,7] The early signs of NF are difficult to detect, and the clinician may be steered toward other less severe diagnoses, including routine postoperative wound cellulitis or hypersensitivity involving the wound or dressing. Laboratory results vary, but are typically consistent with findings of systemic infection (e.g., leukocytosis). Radiographic imaging, including CT or MRI, is insufficient to exclude the diagnosis of NF. Furthermore, the time spent obtaining such imaging may distract from the direct, clinical observation that most commonly leads to timely diagnosis and surgical intervention. Plain films may show subcutaneous air consistent with anaerobic, gas-producing infections, but the absence of visible air on x-ray does not rule out NF.[7]

Other modalities to establish a diagnosis include obtaining a deep-tissue biopsy at the site of inflammation to determine the depth and severity of infection. Typical histopathological findings include aggregation of pathogens at the fascial layer, thrombi, necrosis, polymorphouclear (PMN) infiltrate, and vasculitis.[3] In NF caused by GAS or *S. aureus*, a relative paucity of PMNs owing to leucocidin-mediated destruction has been described.[3] However, such time-consuming diagnostic testing should only be undertaken if the treating clinicians do not already have sufficient evidence for NF to warrant definitive operative management. Most surgeons will prefer surgical exploration as opposed to a bedside biopsy.[7]

Case Presentation (continued)

The surgeon returns to the bedside and finds that the erythema has spread rapidly, more than 3 cm past the margin demarcated by the nurse at the time of her last evaluation. Palpation of the site does not reveal crepitus, but the skin is hot, erythematous, and indurated. The patient is actively rigoring, hypotensive (82/52 mmHg), tachycardic (132 bpm), and febrile (40.2°C). He is disoriented and somnolent. Abdominal exam reveals diffuse, exquisite pain and rebound tenderness on the right. The surgeon immediately calls the operating suite to have a room prepared, telling the scheduler that he plans for an exploratory laparotomy and "debridement of necrotizing fasciitis." He asks the nurse to aggressively administer IV fluids; initiate antibiotic therapy with intravenous vancomycin, clindamycin, and cefepime; and alert the ICU.

Management and Discussion

The decision to proceed immediately to the operating room for management of NF can be life-saving. Antibiotic therapy alone will be insufficient to reverse the course of NF, and mortality approaches 100% in such cases.[7] First, necrotic, devitalized tissue is not well-perfused, even by aggressive dosing of appropriate antimicrobial agents. Second, killing or suppressing bacterial growth alone will not be sufficient because many consequences of NF are mediated by toxins elaborated by the pathogen. Third, surgical exploration will precisely define the extent of infection, confirm the diagnosis, and allow for collection of essential diagnostic cultures. The surgeon must evaluate the extent of necrosis later-ally over the body surface and vertically to be sure deep organ spaces are not involved, especially in the postoperative setting. Operative aerobic and anaerobic tissue cultures are invaluable in determining the primary causative organism(s) and susceptibilities so antimicrobial therapy can be appropriately targeted. Repeated trips to the OR may be necessary to adequately debride and control the extent of the infection, and reexploration within 24 to 48 hours of the initial surgery is recommended.[6,7]

The antimicrobial regimen chosen here is appropriate. Uncertainty about the microbiologic diagnosis and the patient's grave condition warrants broad empiric coverage until additional culture data are available. The emergence of methicillin-resistant *S. aureus* (MRSA) as a cause of aggressive SSTI in both community and hospital settings makes the addition of vancomycin appro-priate, although case reports of monomicrobial MRSA NF are still relatively rare.[8,9] Linezolid or daptomycin may also be used to cover resistant staphylo-cocci. The inclusion of a third- or fourth-generation cephalosporin is appropri-ate given the patient's hospitalization and potential exposure to nosocomial gram negative pathogens, including *P. aeruginosa* or other enterics. A β-lactam/β-lactamase inhibitor (e.g., piperacillin-tazobactam or ticarcillin-clavulanate) or carbapenem (e.g. imipenem) are appropriate alternatives and would also pro-vide the necessary anaerobic coverage.[6]

The inclusion of clindamycin in the regimen goes beyond coverage of anaerobic organisms, which are potential pathogens in this case given recent gastrointestinal surgery. Clindamycin has the additional therapeutic properties of protein synthesis inhibition and toxin suppression, and it has been widely adopted in the management of necrotizing infections and streptococcal toxic shock syndrome.[6] Combination therapy including clindamycin is believed to halt the production of bacterial toxins that are responsible for the rapid spread of infection and limit systemic release of shock-inducing cytokines.[10,11] There is some limited evidence to support this practice both in animal models and observational studies.[6,12,13] Empirically, clindamycin should be used in combina-tion with a β-lactam agent, given the emergence of macrolide resistance in gram positive organisms.[6]

A postoperative case of NF should alert the infection control team at the affected hospital. First, the patient should be placed on contact precautions until draining wounds can be well-contained by a dressing.[14] Second, even a single case of postoperative GAS NF could be considered a "sentinel event" and efforts should be made to identify potential sources of contamination in the perioperative environment and stop any future transmission of this dangerous infection.[3,15] Prior GAS SSI outbreaks have been linked to OR staff members with acute pharyngitis or colonization, and recommendations are available for sampling and decolonization of staff members.[3,15–17]

To date, no specific practices have been definitively linked to an increased risk of subsequent NF after surgery. However, a single devastating episode of NF and source investigation can significantly raise surgical staff members' awareness of the potential for transmitting infections. Such an occurrence can offer a well-timed opportunity to reeducate staff on best practices for SSI prevention in general. These are discussed in detail elsewhere, but recommendations include appropriate and timely perioperative antibiotics, skin preparation, environmental control within the operating room, and strict adherence to sterile technique.[1,2]

Case Conclusion

In the OR, the surgeon discovers copious amounts of dark fluid between the subcutaneous and fascial layers of the abdominal wall and necrosis of the subcutis and fascia without involvement of deeper organs. Extensive debridement is undertaken and the wound is left open to heal. Histopathology shows numerous gram positive organisms in chains. Operative cultures as well as blood cultures grow GAS. The patient goes back to the OR the following day for reexploration and further debridement, and he requires ICU supportive care for 6 days. The patient's antimicrobial regimen is deescalated to cover GAS after initial combination therapy including clindamycin. Over the following weeks, he recovers and is discharged to a rehabilitation center.

Suggested Reading

Anaya DA, Dellinger EP. Necrotizing soft-tissue infection: diagnosis and management. Clin Infect Dis 2007;44(5):705–710.

Morgan MS. Diagnosis and management of necrotising fasciitis: a multiparametric approach. J Hosp Infect 2010;75(4):249–257.

Stevens DL, Bisno AL, Chambers HF, et al. Practice guidelines for the diagnosis and management of skin and soft-tissue infections. Clin Infect Dis 2005;41(10):1373–1406.

References

Anderson DJ, Kaye KS, Classen D, et al. Strategies to prevent surgical site infections in acute care hospitals. Infect Control Hosp Epidemiol 2008;29(Suppl 1):S51–61.

Mangram AJ, Horan TC, Pearson ML, Silver LC, Jarvis WR. Guideline for prevention of surgical site infection, 1999. Hospital Infection Control Practices Advisory Committee. Infect Control Hosp Epidemiol 1999;20(4):250–278; quiz 279–280.

Morgan MS. Diagnosis and management of necrotising fasciitis: a multiparametric approach. J Hosp Infect 2010;75(4):249–257.

Giuliano A, Lewis F, Jr., Hadley K, Blaisdell FW. Bacteriology of necrotizing fasciitis. Am J Surg 1977;134(1):52–57.

de Moya MA, del Carmen MG, Allain RM, Hirschberg RE, Shepard JA, Kradin RL. Case records of the Massachusetts General Hospital. Case 33–2009. A 35-year-old woman with fever, abdominal pain, and hypotension after cesarean section. NEJM 2009;361(17):1689–1697.

Stevens DL, Bisno AL, Chambers HF, et al. Practice guidelines for the diagnosis and management of skin and soft-tissue infections. Clin Infect Dis 2005;41(10):1373–1406.

Anaya DA, Dellinger EP. Necrotizing soft-tissue infection: diagnosis and management. Clin Infect Dis 2007;44(5):705–710.

Young LM, Price CS. Community-acquired methicillin-resistant Staphylococcus aureus emerging as an important cause of necrotizing fasciitis. Surg Infect (Larchmt) 2008;9(4):469–474.

Miller LG, Perdreau-Remington F, Rieg G, et al. Necrotizing fasciitis caused by community-associated methicillin-resistant Staphylococcus aureus in Los Angeles. NEJM 2005;352(14):1445–1453.

Eagle H. Experimental approach to the problem of treatment failure with penicillin. I. Group A streptococcal infection in mice. Am J Med 1952;13(4):389–399.

Stevens DL, Gibbons AE, Bergstrom R, Winn V. The Eagle effect revisited: efficacy of clindamycin, erythromycin, and penicillin in the treatment of streptococcal myositis. J Infect Dis 1988;158(1):23–28.

Zimbelman J, Palmer A, Todd J. Improved outcome of clindamycin compared with beta-lactam antibiotic treatment for invasive Streptococcus pyogenes infection. Pediatr Infect Dis J 1999;18(12):1096–1100.

Mulla ZD, Leaverton PE, Wiersma ST. Invasive group A streptococcal infections in Florida. South Med J 2003;96(10):968–973.

Siegel JD, Rhinehart E, Jackson M, Chiarello L. 2007 Guideline for Isolation Precautions: Preventing Transmission of Infectious Agents in Health Care Settings. Am J Infect Control 2007;35(10 Suppl 2):S65–164.

Prevention of invasive group A streptococcal disease among household contacts of case patients and among postpartum and postsurgical patients: recommendations from the Centers for Disease Control and Prevention. Clin Infect Dis 2002;35(8):950–959.

Ejlertsen T, Prag J, Pettersson E, Holmskov A. A 7-month outbreak of relapsing postpartum group A streptococcal infections linked to a nurse with atopic dermatitis. Scand J Infect Dis 2001;33(10):734–737.

Chan HT, Low J, Wilson L, Harris OC, Cheng AC, Athan E. Case cluster of necrotizing fasciitis and cellulitis associated with vein sclerotherapy. Emerg Infect Dis 2008;14(1):180–181.

Chapter 4b

Varicella Zoster among Hospitalized Patients

Shephali H. Patel and Michael Y. Lin

Initial Case Presentation

A 60 year old woman with newly diagnosed acute leukemia is admitted to the hospital's oncology unit with fever (38.5°C), malaise, and pain in a band-like distribution over the right side of her chest for 1 day. The admitting physician confirms tenderness to touch and mild redness over the right chest. The physician attributes the pain to musculoskeletal strain and prescribes acetaminophen for pain control. The patient is told by the consulting hematologist that she will need to remain hospitalized for further diagnostic tests related to her leukemia and subsequent chemotherapy treatment. Despite this, she feels well enough to leave her room and interact with other patients who are on the ward.

The following day, the patient complains to the nurse about continued right-sided chest pain. Upon examination, the hematologist discovers that numerous vesicles have developed in the area of pain. Some of the vesicles are clear, and others have a cloudy appearance. The rash is one-sided, does not cross the midline, and appears in the skin sensory region of the T4 and T5 nerves (dermatomal distribution).

Differential Diagnosis and Initial Management

Patients who are acutely ill with fever and rash require expedited evaluation from a diagnostic and infection control standpoint because of the risk of transmission of contagion. A key finding is the distribution of the vesicular rash: when it is unilateral and follows a dermatomal pattern. A diagnosis of herpes zoster (commonly referred to as "shingles") can be made based on clinical history and physical examination alone. If the diagnosis is less certain, herpes zoster can be confirmed by submitting vesicular fluid to the lab for any of the following tests: polymerase chain reaction (PCR), direct fluorescent antibody, or viral culture. Other less-likely clinical syndromes that could present in a similar fashion include zosteriform herpes simplex virus, contact dermatitis from allergens such as poison ivy, erysipelas caused by group A streptococci, bullous impetigo, and necrotizing fasciitis. Exceptionally rare but significant causes of vesicles include vaccinia (smallpox vaccine strain) and smallpox (theoretically eradicated but potentially an agent of bioterrorism). Clinical features that distinguish varicella from smallpox are presented in Table 4.2. In this case, the patient's history and physical exam are most consistent with herpes zoster caused by reactivation of varicella zoster virus (VZV). Dermatomal pain can precede the vesicular rash by 2 to 3 days, as observed in this case.

The most infectious member of the herpesvirus family is VZV.[1] Approximately 90% of adults are seropositive for the virus, illustrating its high prevalence and infectivity. The virus produces two distinct clinical syndromes: a primary infection called varicella (chickenpox) and reactivation infection which manifests as herpes zoster (shingles).[2–4]

Varicella (primary VZV infection) affects seronegative persons and typically results in a febrile illness with a disseminated vesicular rash. In a normal host, crops of skin lesions appear over day 2 to 4 of illness, with full crusting of lesions by day 6. Prior to FDA approval of varicella vaccine in 1995, varicella was most commonly seen in children—nearly 90% of American children were infected by age 13. In many developed countries, including the U.S., children are now routinely vaccinated against varicella.

Herpes zoster (reactivation VZV infection) occurs in a subset of individuals who were previously infected with varicella. It typically presents as a painful rash with a dermatomal distribution and affects older adults with waning immunity to varicella zoster virus. The vesicles develop for 3 to 5 days, and total duration of symptoms lasts 10 to 14 days. In some patients, fever, headache, or fatigue accompany the cutaneous findings.

Both varicella and herpes zoster infection, although usually self-limited, can be devastating in the vulnerable hosts commonly encountered in hospitals.[5] Susceptible adults (particularly smokers or pregnant women) who develop varicella are more likely than children to have complications such as pneumonitis. Among immunocompromised hosts, varicella and herpes zoster can be associated with severe complications such as encephalitis, pneumonitis, hepatitis, or secondary bacterial skin and soft tissue infections.[6] Furthermore, varicella

Table 4.2 **Features Distinguishing Varicella (Chickenpox) from Smallpox**
In chickenpox:
No or mild fever prodrome
Lesions are superficial vesicles ("dewdrop on a rose petal").
Lesions appear in crops; on any one part of the body there are lesions in different stages (papules, vesicles, crusts).
Centripetal distribution: greatest concentration of lesions on the trunk, fewest lesions on distal extremities. May involve the face/scalp. Occasionally entire body equally affected.
First lesions appear on the face or trunk.
Palms and soles rarely involved.
Rapid evolution: lesions evolve from macules → papules → vesicles → crusts quickly (<24 hours)
Patients rarely sick or dying.
Patient lacks reliable history of varicella or varicella vaccination.
50%–80% recall an exposure to chickenpox or shingles 10–21 days before rash onset
From http://www.bt.cdc.gov/agent/smallpox/diagnosis/

infection (but not herpes zoster) in VZV-susceptible pregnant women can pre-
cipitate two potentially devastating syndromes for the fetus: congenital varicella
and perinatal varicella. Congenital varicella refers to fetal malformations that
can occur when a susceptible pregnant woman develops primary infection with
the virus. The risk of congenital varicella, less than 2%, is highest in the first half
of pregnancy (up to 20 weeks). Perinatal varicella refers to VZV infection of the
neonate, which can occur if the susceptible mother develops varicella around
the time of delivery. The case mortality associated with neonatal varicella can
be as high as 30%. (Of note, most neonates in hospitals are born to mothers
who are already immune to VZV, and thus are not susceptible to varicella in the
first 6 months of life because of transplacental transfer of protective maternal
antibodies).

Case Presentation (continued)

A sample of the vesicular fluid is tested by PCR and found to be positive for
VZV. Prior to the confirmation of the diagnosis, the patient had not been
placed in contact or airborne precautions. During this time, she had direct contact with several other patients and healthcare workers. One exposed nurse is
pregnant in her third trimester with her first child.

Management and Discussion

Transmission of VZV from person to person occurs via direct skin contact or
via inhalation of virus particles aerosolized from vesicles or respiratory secretions.[7] The virus does not survive well in the environment and is unlikely to be
transmitted on inanimate objects.

Upon acquisition, VZV infects the upper respiratory tract, followed by repli-
cation in the reticuloendothelial system and dissemination via the bloodstream.
The incubation period for varicella (from time of exposure to symptom onset)
is about 14 days for most patients (range, 8–21 days). This relatively long incubation period allows for early serological testing to guide postexposure prophylaxis decisions.

Normal hosts with primary varicella infection are infectious from 1 to 2 days
before until 5 days after the onset of rash. Immunocompromised patients may
be infectious for a longer period of time. Varicella is exceptionally contagious,
with secondary household attack rates as high as 85%. Herpes zoster is also
infectious and a risk for susceptible contacts, although the likelihood of transmission is about one-third that associated with primary varicella. Patients with
herpes zoster are infectious from the time when the vesicular rash emerges
until the rash resolves and the lesions are crusted over. Transmission risk can
be reduced by covering the skin vesicles with clothing or bandages. Herpes zoster is more infectious when disseminated (nonadjacent affected dermatomes or
visceral disease) or in the setting of immunosuppression.

Patients with symptomatic VZV infection require strict adherence to infection control precautions. All patients with primary varicella, disseminated

herpes zoster, or single dermatomal herpes zoster in the setting of immunosuppression should be placed in airborne as well as contact precautions.
Specifically, all individuals entering the patient's hospital room should don
gowns, gloves, and an N-95 respirator. Individuals immune to VZV can theoretically forego an N-95 respirator, although the challenge of ascertaining immune
status, especially among visitors, compels most hospitals to enforce airborne
precautions on an unconditional basis. Patients should be housed in a hospital room that is at negative pressure relative to the adjacent public corridors.
Immunocompetent patients with nondisseminated herpes zoster can be placed
in contact precautions alone. The rash ideally should be covered with clothing
or bandage (Table 4.3).

Of note, nosocomial outbreaks of varicella infection attributed to aerosol
transmission of VZV from immunocompetent patients with localized herpes
zoster have been reported, suggesting that contact precautions without airborne precautions may not be completely sufficient in preventing dissemination. Thus, some hospitals may elect to place all patients with herpes zoster in
both airborne and contact precautions, including immunocompetent patients
with localized herpes zoster.[7]

Once a VZV exposure has occurred in the hospital, hospital infection control staff should immediately initiate an exposure evaluation. Patients, employees, or visitors with significant VZV exposure (defined as being in the same
room or having face-to-face contact with the index patient without adherence
to airborne precautions) must be evaluated. In general, an individual with prior
history of VZV infection (prior varicella, herpes zoster, or vaccination) can be
considered immune, even without further testing. Healthcare workers should
additionally have proof of serologic immunity to VZV, ideally obtained at the
time of employment. If susceptibility status is unclear for any exposed patient
or healthcare worker, VZV serologic testing should be obtained as soon as
possible after the exposure.

Susceptible exposed individuals should be evaluated for postexposure prophylaxis.[8] Healthy susceptible individuals (which would exclude nearly all hospitalized patients) may be provided active immunization with varicella vaccine,
ideally within 5 days of VZV exposure, to prevent subsequent infection or at
least to reduce the severity of clinical manifestations. Passive immunization with

Table 4.3 Isolation Precautions for Hospitalized Patients with Varicella-Zoster Virus Infection

Infection	Isolation precautions
Varicella (primary)	
All	Contact and airborne precautions
Herpes zoster (reactivation)	
Immunocompetent, localized disease	Contact precautions
Immunocompetent, disseminated disease[a]	Contact and airborne precautions
Immunosuppressed, all	Contact and airborne precautions

[a] Disseminated disease refers to herpes zoster occurring in two or more nonadjacent dermatomes, or evidence of visceral disease.

high levels of anti-VZV immunoglobulin (e.g., VariZIG, Cangene Corporation, Winnipeg, Canada) within 96 hours of VZV exposure should be given to exposed individuals with high risk of severe disease (immunosuppressed patients, pregnant women, and newborns whose mother's varicella onset occurred 5 days before to 48 hours after delivery). If VariZIG is not available, IVIG can be used; alternatively, oral acyclovir can be considered for prophylaxis, although the efficacy and optimal dosing for this approach are unclear.

Exposed susceptible individuals should be observed for symptoms and signs of varicella from days 8 to 21 postexposure (for individuals receiving anti-VZV immunoglobulin, days 8 to 28, because passive immunization may delay the onset of clinical disease).[8] Exposed susceptible patients need to be placed in airborne precautions during the observation period, with contact precautions initiated if varicella occurs. Exposed susceptible healthcare workers should be furloughed from patient care during the observation period.

Treatment of hospitalized patients with either varicella or herpes zoster is aimed at reducing complications, improving symptoms, and shortening duration of illness and infectivity. Treatment should be initiated early in the course of disease for optimal efficacy. Acyclovir is approved for treatment of both varicella and herpes zoster, and is available orally and intravenously. Valacyclovir is an oral prodrug of acyclovir with superior systemic absorption; it is approved for treatment of herpes zoster in healthy individuals. Both require dose adjustment for kidney insufficiency.

Individuals developing varicella who are at risk for complications (for example, children with skin or lung disease; additionally, all adolescents and adults) should be treated with antiviral therapy within 24 hours of symptom onset.[3] In contrast, treatment of varicella in healthy children is optional given the low risk of serious disease and complications. For healthy children 2 to 16 years old, oral dosage is 20 mg/kg four times daily for 5 days, with a maximum of 800 mg daily; healthy adolescents and adults receive acyclovir 800 mg orally, five times daily, for 5 to 7 days. All immune compromised individuals with varicella should be treated with intravenous acyclovir (10 mg/kg every 8 hours for 7 days) rather than oral acyclovir, regardless of time from onset of symptoms, to prevent complications.

All patients with herpes zoster are generally treated to hasten recovery and prevent postherpetic neuralgia. Treatment of herpes zoster is similar to that of varicella with the exceptions that treatment duration is typically longer (7–10 days) and valacyclovir is often preferred over oral acyclovir for this indication. Immune compromised individuals with disseminated herpes zoster should receive intravenous acyclovir, while those with localized disease can be treated with either oral or intravenous antiviral therapy.

Case Conclusion

The index patient in this case had localized herpes zoster (adjacent dermatomes) but was immune compromised because of her leukemia. Therefore, she was placed in airborne and contact precautions and given intravenous acyclovir for treatment. The hospital infection control staff started an exposure evaluation that revealed that three other patients and two nurses (one of whom was pregnant) had significant contact. The exposed patients had unknown VZV history and thus were tested for VZV serology, two of whom were found to be susceptible. One patient (immunocompetent) was placed in airborne precautions for days 8 to 21 post exposure; a second patient (immunosuppressed) was given VariZIG and placed in airborne precautions for days 8 to 28 postexposure. One exposed nurse (pregnant) was found to have prior documented immunity to VZV. As such, no further action was taken and she continued to work. A second exposed nurse (healthy, non-pregnant) had an unknown VZV immune status. She was tested and found to be serologically negative for VZV. She was given varicella vaccine by the third postexposure day and was furloughed from work for days 8 to 21 postexposure. No secondary varicella cases occurred among any exposed individuals.

References

Arvin AM. Varicella-zoster virus. Clin Microbiol Rev 1996;9(3):361–381.

Gnann JW Jr, Whitley RJ. Clinical practice. Herpes zoster. NEJM 2002; 347(5):340–346.

Whitley RJ. Varicella-Zoster Virus. In: Mandell GL, Bennett JE, Dolin R, eds. Principles and practice of infectious diseases. Philadelphia: Churchill Livingstone, 2010:1963–1969.

Straus SE, Ostrove JM, Inchauspe G, et al. NIH conference. Varicella-zoster virus infections. Biology, natural history, treatment, and prevention. Ann Intern Med 1988;108(2):221–237.

Gnann JW, Jr. Varicella-zoster virus: atypical presentations and unusual complications. J Infect Dis 2002;186(Suppl 1):S91–98.

Feldman S, Hughes WT, Daniel CB. Varicella in children with cancer: Seventy-seven cases. Pediatrics 1975;56(3):388–397.

Weber DJ, Rutala WA, Hamilton H. Prevention and control of varicella-zoster infections in healthcare facilities. Infect Control Hosp Epidemiol 1996;17(10):694–705.

Siegel JD, Rhinehart E, Jackson M, Chiarello L. 2007 Guideline for isolation precautions: preventing transmission of infectious agents in health care settings. Am J Infect Control 2007;35(10 Suppl 2):S65–164.

Chapter 4c

Scabies, Bedbugs and other Infestations in the Hospital

Maureen Bolon

Initial Case Presentation

A 67-year-old woman is admitted to an inpatient medicine unit from a nursing home for an exacerbation of congestive heart failure. She is treated with aggressive diuresis and a new cardiac ischemic event is excluded. By the third day of hospitalization her presenting symptoms of dyspnea on exertion and orthopnea have improved. During morning rounds she reports bothersome itching and requests that she be prescribed a "pill, ointment or cream" to give her some relief. Upon further questioning the patient reports that she in fact has had a several week history of itching, predominantly involving her hands, wrists, and bilateral underarms. The itching has been keeping her awake at night. On examination of her skin she is found to have excoriations involving her upper extremities and axillae. A few erythematous papules are noted in the axillae and several gray markings that appear to be beneath the skin surface are noted on her right wrist. Her medication list is reviewed without identifying a likely contributor to the pruritis. An oral antihistamine is prescribed for the itching and a consulting dermatologist is asked to see the patient.

Differential Diagnosis and Initial Management

Although there are numerous possible etiologies of a pruritic rash in a hospitalized patient, several features of this case should lead the clinician to suspect scabies. Intense pruritis that is particularly troublesome at night is a hallmark of classical scabies, which often affects individuals who live in institutional settings such as a nursing home, as was the case for this patient. Manifestations of the rash can vary, but linear burrows, which are gray or pigmented lines up to a centimeter in length, and erythematous papules or nodules, are most commonly observed. Lesions typically occur in the finger webs, wrists, elbows, axillae, breasts, periumbilical area, genitals, buttocks, and knees.

The causative agent of scabies is the mite *Sarcoptes scabiei* var. *hominus*. Humans are the primary reservoir for *S. scabiei*, an ovoid arthropod that cannot be visualized with the naked eye. The pathognomonic burrow of scabies is caused by the tunneling of the female mite into the stratum corneum in order to lay eggs. A definitive diagnosis of scabies requires a skin scraping to recover mites, mite feces, or eggs that are identified microscopically. Mites are typically not recovered from scabeous papules or nodules, because these manifestations of infestation are a result of host hypersensitivity reaction. Scabies mites are not thought to transmit other infectious diseases through their bites; however, secondary bacterial infection caused by group A streptococcus or *Staphylococcus aureus* is a potential complication of broken skin caused by scratching.

A severe and potentially life-threatening presentation of scabies known as crusted scabies (formerly Norwegian scabies) should be mentioned. Crusted scabies most typically affects individuals with depressed immune systems. Skin lesions in these cases are best described as thick and scaly plaques that may involve any part of the body (Fig. 4.1). Lymphadenopathy and eosinophilia may also accompany the skin findings. Surprisingly, pruritis is not a predominant symptom of crusted scabies. The resultant failure to kill the mites by scratching is one factor that accounts for the very high burden of organisms in these cases. Individuals with crusted scabies may harbor as many as several million mites, whereas patients with classical infestation typically only harbor ten to twelve mites. In general, a suspected diagnosis of crusted scabies should prompt hospital admission.

Bedbugs have recently resurged as a concern in the developed world. Otherwise known as *Cimex lectularius*, the bedbug is a nighttime-biter and like scabies causes an itchy rash. Individuals suffering with bedbug bites may share some of the same risk factors as those with scabies infestation, namely crowded living conditions or institutional residence. However, numerous distinctions

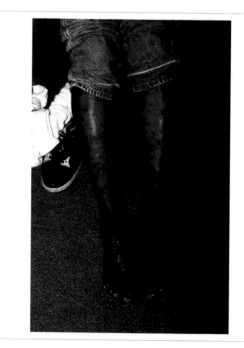

Figure 4.1 Crusted scabies in a patient with HIV infection.

must be made between these infestations (Table 4.4). *C. lectularius* is a reddish-brown arthropod that is visible with the naked eye, unlike the much smaller *S. scabei*. Bedbugs do not reside on humans, but rather live in their environment, travelling to the slumbering human as their main food source and then returning to dwell in tiny cracks and crevices in furniture and walls after a blood meal. Bedbug bites resemble those of other biting insects: manifesting as small, pruritic, erythematous papules or macules 2 to 5 millimeters in diameter. Individuals with a robust immune response may experience larger wheals. Bites are typically distributed in a line or curve on unclothed skin following the bedbug's traverse. Although bites may be complicated by secondary bacterial infection,

Table 4.4 Comparison of the Features of Infestation with Scabies Versus Bedbugs

Feature	Scabies	Bedbugs
Causative organism	*Sarcoptes scabiei* var. *hominis*	*Cimex lectularius*
Description of organism	Ovoid with a small anterior cephalic and a caudal thoraco-abdominal portion. Ranges in size from 0.3–0.4 mm	Reddish-brown, flat, wingless oval arthropod. Ranges in size from 4–7 mm
Habitat	Obligate human parasite	Human environment Bat or bird roosts
Life span	30–60 days	6–12 months
Duration of survival between feedings	2–3 days	12 months to 2 years (bedbugs may live longer between feedings in colder climates)
Method of transmission	Classical scabies: direct skin-to-skin contact between 15–20 minutes duration Crusted scabies: direct contact and potential for transmission via infested skin squames shed into the environment	Active dispersal: bedbugs can walk short distances (5–20 feet) within a room for a blood meal. Passive dispersal: bedbugs can travel long distances by being transported by humans in clothing, luggage, or furniture.
Vector of human disease	No	No
Comparison of clinical manifestations of scabies and bedbugs		
Feature	Scabies	Bedbugs
Typical appearance of rash	Intensely pruritic linear burrows with a small pearl-like vesicle at one end. Violaceous, pruritic nodules and papules.	A line of several 2–5 mm pruritic papules or macules. May have a central hemorrhagic punctum at the bite site.
Less common appearance of rash	Crusted scabies: hyperkeratotic dermatosis resembling psoriasis, crusted plaques, commonly involves the nails.	Wheals several centimeters in size, purpuric lesions, vesicular lesions, bullous lesions
Distribution of bites	Finger webs, flexor surfaces, breasts, belt line, genitals	Skin exposed while sleeping
Accompanying symptoms	Lymphadenopathy, eosinophilia (in crusted scabies)	Anemia, asthma, anaphylaxis (all rare)

extensive investigation has failed to implicate bedbugs as a vector of any infectious illness. Beyond the characteristics of the rash, the best way to establish a diagnosis of bedbug infestation is to demonstrate evidence of infestation in the patient's home environment. Such evidence may include visualization of the insect, insect excrement, or blood spots on the mattress or bed linen. Crevices in the vicinity of the bed, such as in box springs, bed frames, headboards, baseboards, or picture frames may also display signs of bedbug activity.

Case Presentation (continued)

The consulting Dermatologist confirms a diagnosis of classical scabies after examining a scraping of the patient's skin. She is placed in contact isolation until she completes treatment with topical permethrin cream. The patient's daughter, who was her primary caretaker until the recent admission to a nursing home, asks whether any family members should be tested for scabies. Several nurses on the medicine ward who cared for her before her diagnosis was recognized also request evaluation for scabies.

Management and Discussion

Although there are several topical agents that have been used to treat scabies, permethrin is believed to be the most effective option. Permethrin is administered as a 5% cream that is applied to the entire surface of the skin and washed off after 8 to 12 hours. A second dose should be similarly applied 1 week after the first. Permethrin acts on sodium channels in the mite, causing paralysis and death, but has minimal toxicity in humans. Potential side effects in humans are related to skin irritation. Patients should be reevaluated 4 weeks after any form of treatment to ensure eradication of the mites.

One other therapeutic option that should be noted is the oral medication, ivermectin. This agent has been used extensively against parasitic diseases in the developing world and is also effective against the scabies mite. The primary use of ivermectin is as an adjunct to topical therapy when treating crusted scabies. It may also be chosen for treatment of contacts of scabies cases because of its relative ease of use compared to topical medications. It is administered as an oral dose of 200 mg, followed by a repeat dose in 14 days to kill any mites that may have hatched after the original dose.

Scabies is well-known for causing infestation among household contacts and within healthcare institutions, thus evaluation and treatment of any individual with prolonged close contact with the index case is warranted. Yet again, it is helpful to differentiate between classical scabies and crusted scabies, which present markedly different risk to contacts. In classical scabies, the low organism burden serves as an impediment to widespread transmission. Prolonged skin to skin contact is required for transmission, because it can take several minutes for a mite to penetrate human skin. In contrast, the very high mite burden characteristic of crusted scabies facilitates transmission to even casual contacts. Additionally, because mites are shed into the environment in great quantities from cases of crusted scabies, transmission via fomites such as clothing, bedding, and furniture becomes a concern. Outbreaks within healthcare institutions involving both patients and healthcare workers have been reported following unrecognized cases of crusted scabies. In addition to prescribing topical or oral therapy to all known contacts of the index case (preferably by treating case and contacts simultaneously to prevent re-infestation), a very systematic approach to case identification and environmental disinfection must be pursued. For patients with scabies who require nonelective surgery, procedures can be performed with the use of contact precautions (gown & glove) and thorough cleaning of the operating room following the procedure.

Because bedbugs do not infest humans, but rather their environment, there is no specific therapy required for patients presenting with evidence of bedbug bites. Pruritis is typically treated symptomatically with topical corticosteroids and oral antihistamines. Evaluation and monitoring for secondary bacterial infection is reasonable, particularly in cases with marked skin excoriation. There is minimal risk of transmission of bedbugs to healthcare workers, even those with close contact. However, in settings in which patients bring luggage or other potentially infested belongings from home, a very thorough inspection and cleaning of the environment may be warranted following patient discharge in order to prevent infestation of the hospital room. Hospital gowns and bed linens may be laundered in the usual manner. Bedbug eradication in the home environment is best left to those with pest management experience.

Case Conclusion

The patient reports continued itching following her treatment with permethrin cream, which is repeated at 7 days as planned. In the absence of further evidence of active scabies infestation, the prolonged pruritis is considered a consequence of her immune reaction to the infestation. This is managed symptomatically and gradually subsides. Her family members receive preventive treatment with permethrin as do two nurses and three patient care technicians who reported close contact with the patient prior to the identification of the scabies. Her clothing and bedding are laundered and items that cannot be laundered are stored in impermeable plastic bags for 10 days to ensure mite death. The nursing home where she resided prior to admission is also informed of the potential for scabies infestation and conducts an independent investigation. No further cases of scabies are reported in the hospital in the subsequent weeks.

Suggested Reading

Bouvresse S, Chosidow O. Scabies in healthcare settings. Curr Opin Infect Dis 2010;23:111–118.

Goddard J, deShazo R. Bed bugs (Cimex lectularius) and clinical consequences of their bites. JAMA 2009;301:1358–1366.

Delaunay P, Blanc V, Del Giudice P, et al. Bedbugs and infectious diseases. Clin Infect Dis 2011;52:200–210.

Hicks MI, Elston DM. Scabies. Dermatol Ther 2009;22:279–92.

Strong M, Johnstone PW. Interventions for treating scabies. Cochrane Database Syst Rev 2007:CD000320.

Chapter 4d

Prosthetic Joint Infection

Evgenia Kagan and Camelia Marculescu

A 58-year-old man with morbid obesity, type II diabetes mellitus, and recurrent facial folliculitis underwent a right total knee arthroplasty for osteoarthritis 2 months prior to admission. He initially did well, but at the time of his suture removal a local hematoma was noted. Three weeks after surgery, he developed sudden onset of knee swelling, fever up to 101°F, and pain. He was evaluated by his primary care physician and prescribed a 10-day course of cephalexin with mild improvement of his symptoms; however, he eventually presented to the hospital where on exam, a swollen knee was noted with mild sanguineous discharge. Plain radiographs of the knee revealed a well-seated prosthesis with a small effusion in the joint space. Peripheral white blood cell count was normal. Sedimentation rate (ESR) was 53 mm/h, and low sensitivity C-reactive protein (CRP) was 2.3mg/dl. The joint aspirate fluid showed 43,000 WBC with 93% neutrophils. Gram stain did not reveal microorganisms and initial bacterial cultures were negative.

The number of joint replacement surgeries has increased every year for decades and it is estimated that the number of total knee arthroplasties performed by 2030 will be 3.48 million. Infections associated with prosthetic joints account for significant morbidity and can lead to poor functional outcome and rarely death. In patients undergoing primary joint replacement, infection rates for common procedures are less than 1% for hip and shoulder prostheses, less than 2% for knee prostheses, and less than 9% for elbow prostheses; However, infection rates among patients undergoing revision procedures are reportedly as high as 20%.

Several risk factors for prosthetic joint infection (PJI), such as rheumatoid arthritis, psoriasis, immunosuppression, steroid therapy, poor nutritional status, obesity, diabetes mellitus, and advanced age of 70 years or older have been reported in case series. The presence of a malignancy and history of previous joint arthroplasty have been associated with an increased risk of PJI in case control studies. The patient described has diabetes mellitus and obesity as risk factors.

Inoculation of microorganisms into the surgical wound may occur periop-eratively (during surgery or immediately thereafter), may be spread hematog-enously from a distant focus of infection, or occur contiguously (spreading from an adjacent focus of infection). These infections can present as super-ficial cellulitis, abscess, or deep-seated infection. According to the onset of symptoms after implantation, PJI are classified as early (those that develop less than 3 months after surgery), usually caused by highly virulent organisms (e.g., *Staphylococcus aureus* or gram-negative bacilli; delayed 3 to 24 months after surgery), generally caused by less virulent organisms (e.g., coagulase-negative staphylococci or *Propionibacterium acnes*); and late (more than 24 months after surgery) predominantly caused by hematogenous seeding from a remote focus of infection. Acute onset of fever, joint pain, effusion, erythema, and warmth at the implant site within a few weeks after surgery suggest an early infection in our patient.

During the course of infection, clinically significant cellulitis and formation of a sinus tract with purulent discharge may occur. Patients with delayed infec-tion usually present with more subtle signs and symptoms, such as implant loosening, persistent joint pain, or both, which may be difficult to distinguish from aseptic failure. Often a combination of preoperative and intraoperative tests is necessary for accurate diagnosis. Peripheral blood leukocyte count with differential may remain normal even in the presence of infection. After sur-gery, CRP is usually elevated and returns to normal within weeks. Repetitive measurements establishing a pattern with clinical correlation are often more informative than a single value.

Synovial fluid analysis is a simple, rapid, and accurate test for differentiating infection from aseptic failure. It is important to recognize that the leukocyte count and differential cut-off values for diagnosing PJI are considerably lower than those for diagnosing septic arthritis in native joints. In patients without underlying inflammatory joint disease, a synovial-fluid leukocyte count of more than 1700 per cubic millimeter or a finding of more than 65 percent neutrophils has sensitivities for infection of 94% and 97%, respectively, and specificities of 88% and 98%, respectively. A high leukocyte count with neutrophilic predomi-nance was evident in the joint aspirate of our patient.

Histopathological Diagnosis

Finding 1 to 10 or more neutrophils per high-power field at a magnification of 400 on histopathological examination has a sensitivity of more than 80 percent and a specificity of more than 90 percent for the presence of infection, but interobserver variability is also high.

Microbiological Diagnosis

Gram staining of synovial fluid and periprosthetic tissue has a high specificity (more than 97%) but generally a low sensitivity (less than 26%). Therefore, a negative result is often unreliable and adds little value to the diagnosis of PJI. Cultures of periprosthetic tissue provide the most reliable means of detecting the pathogen. Positive cultures of the aspirated synovial fluid reported in case series range from 45% to 100%. At least three intraoperative tissue specimens should be sampled for culture. Culturing of a superficial wound or sinus tract should generally be avoided as they are often positive because of microbial colonization from the surrounding skin. Cultures may be negative owing to prior antimicrobial exposure, a low number of or the presence of fastidious organisms, an inappropriate culture medium, or a prolonged transport time to the microbiology laboratory. To detect cases of low-grade infection (infection which typically presents only with early loosening of the prosthesis and persistent pain, often without systemic or local clinical signs of infection), antimicrobial therapy should be discontinued at least two weeks before tissue specimens are obtained.

Radiographic Diagnosis

Plain radiographs are often helpful to diagnose infection especially when they are studied serially over time after implantation. Prosthesis loosening, new subperiosteal bone growth, and transcortical sinus tracts are specific for infection (Fig. 4.2). However, migration of the implant and periprosthetic osteolysis can also occur without infection. Arthrography is useful for detecting implant loosening, pseudobursae, and abscesses.

In several studies, infection was diagnosed if at least one of the following criteria was present: growth of the same microorganism in two or more cultures of synovial fluid or periprosthetic tissue, purulence of synovial fluid at the implant site, acute inflammation on histopathological examination of periprosthetic tissue, or presence of a sinus tract communicating with the prosthesis.

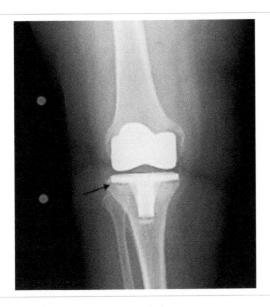

Figure 4.2 Chronic TKA infection with loose tibial component.

(Reproduced with permission from Yoshikawa T, Norman D. Infectious disease in the aging: a clinical handbook, 2nd ed. New York: Humana Press, 2009.)

Case Presentation (continued)

The patient was taken to the OR and underwent debridement of the knee joint with retention of the prosthesis and exchange of the polyethylene liner. All three intraoperative cultures of periprosthetic tissue grew methicillin-resistant *Staphylococcus aureus* (MRSA) with a vancomycin MIC of 1 mcg/ml (microdilution technique). The isolate was resistant to erythromycin and moxifloxacin, and susceptible to trimethoprim/sulfamethoxazole, clindamycin, tetracycline, linezolid, and daptomycin.

The patient was successfully treated with intravenous vancomycin plus rifampin for 6 weeks, followed by oral therapy with trimethoprim-sulfamethoxazole plus rifampin for an additional 14 weeks. Use of vancomycin requires knowledge of dosing parameters and selection of target trough levels appropriate to the specific infection and to the pathogen being treated. For clinicians, it is essential to remain up-to-date with evolving definitions for vancomycin susceptibility, with new interpretations of efficacy and toxicity. The trough vancomycin serum concentration should be greater than 10 mg/l to prevent the development of resistance, and trough levels of 15 to 20 mg/l are recommended if the minimum inhibitory concentration (MIC) is 1 mg/l or higher.

Management

Successful treatment of PJI requires adequate surgical debridement combined with long-term antimicrobial therapy. The goal of treatment is to cure the infection and improve the functional outcome. Medical treatment alone may be justified in patients at high risk for intraoperative or postoperative complications. In this instance lifelong antibiotic suppressive therapy is often required.

Different surgical modalities may be utilized: debridement with retention of prosthesis; a one-stage exchange (the infected prosthesis is removed and a new one implanted in the same procedure); resection arthroplasty and delayed reimplantation (two-stage exchange); resection arthroplasty with or without arthrodesis, and amputation. Zimmerli et al. developed a treatment algorithm which was validated in cohort studies with an overall success rate of more than 80% (Figs. 4.3 and 4.4).

Antimicrobial therapy is given according to the susceptibility pattern of the pathogen. Empiric antibiotic therapy may be indicated in the rare instance in which a patient with PJI presents with sepsis, complicated soft tissue infection, or is otherwise unstable to await culture and sensitivity results. In general, antimicrobial therapy should be withheld for at least 10 to 14 days prior to the culture ascertainment at the time of surgical debridement to ensure adequate growth of microorganisms. In staphylococcal infections, rifampin has activity for surface-adhering, slow-growing, and biofilm-producing microorganisms; however, rifampin should never be used as monotherapy because of rapid development of resistance. Suggested antimicrobial therapy is summarized in Table 4.5.

Our patient had MRSA isolated from the periprosthetic tissue. Vancomycin is generally the drug of choice to treat such infections; however, successful outcomes of therapies with vancomycin for MRSA PJI have been inversely

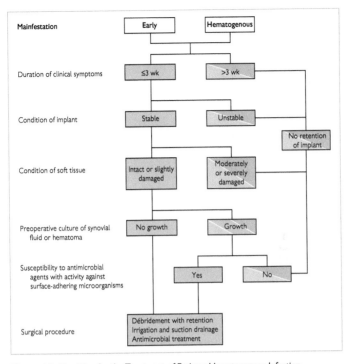

Figure 4.3 Algorithm for the Treatment of Early or Hematogenous Infection
Associated with a Prosthetic Joint
This algorithm can be used for the treatment of patients with various types of arthroplasties; however, it has been used most frequently with patients who have hip and knee
arthroplasties.

(Reproduced with permission from Zimmerli W, Trampuz A, Ochsner PE. Prosthetic-joint infections.
NEJM 2004;351:1645–1654.)

correlated to the vancomycin minimum inhibitory concentration. For bacteremia, MRSA isolates with vancomycin MICs less than 0.5 µg/ml have been
successfully treated with vancomycin 55.6% of the time but isolates with higher
MICs (> 1 to 2 µg/ml) have much lower success rates, with some reports of less
than 10%. The implications of an increased vancomycin MIC when treating musculoskeletal infections is not well understood. Several alternative antimicrobials
with activity against MRSA include linezolid, daptomycin, trimethoprim–sul-
famethoxazole, or tigecycline. Optimal duration of treatment of PJI is not standardized. Zimmerli et al. have suggested treatment duration for 3 months for
hip prostheses and six months for knee prostheses.

In summary, when treating PJI, one must consider the type of infection, the
virulence, and antimicrobial susceptibilities of the microorganism(s) involved,
side effects of antimicrobial therapy, alternative options, and condition of the
host. The administration of systemic antimicrobial therapy should be done
under the guidance of an infectious disease specialist in close collaboration with
the orthopedic surgeon caring for these patients.

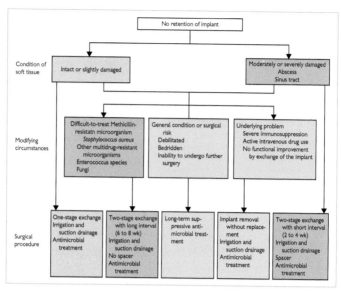

Figure 4.4 Algorithm for the Treatment of Patients with Infections Not Qualifying for Implant Retention

This algorithm has been developed for patients with a hip prosthesis who have delayed or late infection, symptoms of more than 3 weeks duration, for patients with a hip prosthesis who have delayed or late infection with difficult-to-treat microorganisms, severely compromised soft tissue, or a severe coexisting illness. In patients with a knee prosthesis, arthrodesis is performed after resection arthroplasty. If the soft tissue is intact or only slightly damaged, a one-stage exchange (*green boxes*) may be possible. In patients with compromised soft tissue or difficult-to-treat microorganisms, a two-stage exchange (*blue boxes*) is preferred. Permanent explantation or joint arthrodesis is usually performed in severely immunocompromised patients, those with active intravenous drug use, and those in whom arthroplasty will not provide any functional benefit (*gray boxes*).

(Reproduced with permission from Zimmerli W, Trampuz A, Ochsner PE. Prosthetic-joint infections. NEJM 2004;351:1645–1654.)

Prevention of PJI

There are several infection control initiatives designed to prevent MRSA transmission in acute care settings that have gained considerable support in the past decade. The MRSA prevention interventions include: (1) use of systems and behavioral change strategies to promote adherence to infection control protocol, (2) enhanced emphasis on hand hygiene and environmental disinfection, (3) active surveillance testing of anterior nares and open wounds within 48 hours after admission to identify patients symptomatically colonized with MRSA for prompt initiation of contact precautions, and (4) MRSA decolonization (using intranasal mupirocin and chlorhexidine bathing).

Use of perioperative systemic antimicrobial prophylaxis is recommended to reduce the microbial inoculum that may be introduced into the surgical site at the time of surgery. It is directed against the microorganisms most likely

Table 4.5 Suggested Antimicrobial Therapy for Selected Microorganisms in Adult Patients with PJI[a]

Microorganism	First choice	Second line
Staphylococcus spp. Methicillin-susceptible	Nafcillin sodium 1.5–2 g IV q4 h or Cefazolin, 1–2 g IV q8 h	Vancomycin 15 mg/kg IV q12 h or Levofloxacin, 500–750 mg PO or IV q24 h + rifampin, 300–450 po q12 h[b]
Staphylococcus spp. Methicillin-resistant	Vancomycin, 15 mg/kg IV q12 h	Linezolid, 600 mg PO or IV q12 h or Levofloxacin, 500–750 mg PO or IV q24 h + rifampin, 300–450 mg PO q 12 h[b]
Enterococcus spp. penicillin-susceptible[c]	Aqueous crystalline penicillin G, 20–24 million units IV q24 h continuously or in six divided doses or Ampicillin sodium, 12 g IV q24 h continuously or in six divided doses	Vancomycin, 15 mg/kg IV q12 h
Enterococcus spp. penicillin-resistant[c]	Vancomycin, 15 mg/kg IV q12h	Linezolid, 600 mg PO or IV q12h
Pseudomonas aeruginosa[d]	Cefepime, 1–2 g IV q12 h or Meropenem, 1 g IV q8 h or Imipenem, 500 mg IV q6–8 h	Ciprofloxacin, 750 mg PO or 400 mg IV q12 h or Ceftazidime, 2 g IV q8 h
Enterobacter spp.	Meropenem, 1 g IV q8 h or Imipenem, 500 mg IV q6–8 h	Cefepime, 1–2 g IV q12 h or Ciprofloxacin, 750 mg PO or 400 mg IV q12 h
beta-hemolytic streptococci	Aqueous crystalline penicillin G, 20–24 million units IV q24 h by continuous infusion or in six divided doses or Ceftriaxone, 1–2 g IV q24 h	Vancomycin, 15 mg/kg IV q12 h
Propionibacterium acnes and Corynebacterium spp	Aqueous crystalline penicillin G, 20–24 IV q24 h by continuous infusion or in six divided doses or Ceftriaxone 1–2 g IV q24 h or Vancomycin, 15 mg/kg IV q12 h	Clindamycin, 600–900 mg IV q8 mg h

[a] Dose based on normal renal and hepatic function may need to be adjusted if renal or hepatic impairment exists. Recommendations assume in vitro susceptibility and no allergies.

[b] Levofloxacin–rifampin combination therapy for patients managed by debridement with retention. If organism susceptible to levofloxacin, cotrimoxazole or minocycline may be substituted. Rifampin would also be used in combination with the intravenous therapy as well if treating a PJI that has been managed with debridement and retention.

[c] Addition of aminoglycoside for bactericidal synergy is optional. Considerations in choice of an agent are similar to those noted for treatment of enterococcal endocarditis.

[d] Addition of an aminoglycoside is optional.

Modified with permission from Sia IG, Berbari EF, Karchmer AW. Prosthetic joint infections. Infect Dis Clin North Am2005;19(4):885–814.

to contaminate the surgical wound. Cefazolin has specifically been shown to reduce the risk of PJI. Alternatively, cefuroxime may be used as prophylaxis. For patients with severe ß-lactam or known cephalosporin allergies, prophylaxis with vancomycin or clindamycin is recommended. Use of vancomycin prophylaxis is also recommended under certain circumstances, such as known outbreaks of infection due to MRSA, high endemic rates of surgical site infection due to MRSA, high-risk patients such as those with diabetes, and high-risk procedures during which an implant is placed.

In addition to prevention strategies targeting procedure-related issues such as antimicrobial-loaded bone cement placement, there are also a number of prevention strategies that focus on modifiable patient-related risk factors for surgical site infection. These include preoperative blood glucose control for patients with diabetes and minimizing use of immunosuppressive medications whenever possible. For obese patients, appropriate dosing of perioperative systemic antimicrobials is very important.

Case Conclusion

The patient was seen in follow-up 6 months after surgery and continues to do well. He is without signs or symptoms of recurrent infection and has good functionality of the prosthetic joint.

Suggested Reading

Atkins BL, Athanasou N, Deeks JJ, et al. Prospective evaluation of criteria for microbiological diagnosis of prosthetic-joint infection at revision arthroplasty. J Clin Microbiol 1998;36:2932–2939.

Berbari EF, Hanssen AD, Duffy MC, Steckelberg JM, Ilstrup DM, Harmsen WS, et al. Risk factors for prosthetic joint infections: case control study. Clin Infect Dis 1998; 27(5):1247–1254.

Lentino JR. Prosthetic joint infections: bane of orthopedists, challenge for infectious disease specialists. Clin Infect Dis 2003;36(9):1157–1161.

Marculescu CE, Berbari EF, Hanssen AD, Steckelberg JM, Harmsen SW, Mandrekar JN, et al. Outcome of prosthetic joint infections treated with debridement and retention of components. Clin Infect Dis 2006;42(4):471–478.

Osmon DR, Hanssen AD, Patel R . Prosthetic joint infection: Criteria for future definitions. Clin Orthop Relat Res 2005;437:89–90.

Sakoulas G, Moise-Broder PA, Schentag J, Forrest A, Moellering RC Jr., Eliopoulos GM. Relationship of MIC and bactericidal activity to efficacy of vancomycin for treatment of methicillin-resistant Staphylococcus aureus bacteremia. J Clin Microbiol 2004;42(6):2398–2402.

Sia IG , Berbari EF , Karchmer AW. Prosthetic joint infections. Infect Dis Clin North Am 2005;19(4):885–914.

Steckelberg JM, Osmon DR. Prosthetic joint infection. In: Bisno AL, Waldvogel FA, eds. Infections associiated with indwelling medical devices, 3rd ed. Washington, DC: American Society of Microbioly, 2000:173–209.

Trampuz A, Hanssen AD, Osmon DR, Mandrekar J, Steckelberg JM, Patel R. Synovial fluid leukocyte count and differential for the diagnosis of prosthetic knee infection. Am J Med 2004; 117:556–562.

Trampuz A, Steckelberg JM, Osmon DR, Cockerill FR, Hanssen AD, Patel R. Advances in the laboratory diagnosis of prosthetic joint infection. Rev Med Microbiol 2003;14:1–14.

Trampuz A, Zimmerli W. Prosthetic joint infections: update in diagnosis and treatment. Swiss Med Wkly 2005;135(17–18):243–251.

Zimmerli W, Trampuz A, Ochsner PE. Prosthetic-joint infections. NEJM 2004;351:1645–1654.

Chapter 5a

Healthcare-Associated *Clostridium difficile* Infection

Carlene A. Muto

Case Presentation

An 84-year-old woman presented to the Emergency Department with a 2-day history of diarrhea. One month prior she was diagnosed with necrotizing fasciitis of the left lower extremity due to *Strep pyogenes*. This required multiple surgical debridements and intravenous antibiotics of nafcillin and clindamycin. Clindamycin was discontinued after 1 week and she completed a 2-week course of nafcillin. On presentation she admitted to 10 watery bowel movements per day, abdominal pain and nausea but no vomiting. She noted tactile fevers. She denied weight loss or bloody stool. She had no sick contacts, denied travel, and had not eaten outside her home. Other medical history is only significant for peptic ulcer disease for which she takes an over the counter proton pump inhibitor.

On examination the patient was awake but disoriented. Temperature was 101.5°F, pulse 122 per minute, respiratory rate of 24 per minute and blood pressure of 90/55. She had lower quadrant tenderness and abdominal distention. Bowel sounds were absent. The surgical site was without erythema or discharge. Lab values revealed a white blood cell count of 49,500 (55% neutrophils, 40% bands), liver function tests were normal, albumin was 2.1, creatinine was 2.5 (1.3 last admission), and serum lactate was 5.5. CT scan of the abdomen and pelvis revealed diffuse colitis and stool testing confirmed toxigenic *Clostridium difficile* (*C. diff*).

Differential Diagnosis and Initial Management

The differential diagnosis for this febrile diarrheal illness includes both viral causes of acute gastroenteritis such as Norovirus and Rotavirus, as well as the invasive enteric pathogens *Escherichia Coli, Shigella, Salmonella, Campylobacter, Yersinia, Aeromonas,* and *Plesiomonas,* and *C. diff*. Presence of fever and lack of vomiting make viral gastroenteritis and some enteric pathogens less likely and a positive stool test for *C. diff* suggests this is the cause. Risk factors for *Clostridium difficile* infection (CDI) include recent hospitalization, receipt of antibiotics, advanced age, and proton pump inhibitor use. Her history and clinical exam were significant for common features of CDI such as frequent watery diarrhea (often up to 20 stools per day) abdominal pain, tenderness, and distension. Absence of bowel sounds may indicate severe disease complicated by toxic megacolon. Fever and mental status changes also suggest moderate or severe disease. The patient's laboratory findings were consistent with severe CDI (leukocytosis with bandemia, renal insufficiency, hypoalbuminemia, and elevated lactate).

Despite fluid resuscitation, blood pressure remained low, thus vasopressor therapy was initiated. The patient was treated with IV metronidazole and oral vancomycin via a nasogastric tube. She was admitted to the intensive care unit where she remained febrile with increasing abdominal pain. WBC remained elevated and lactate continued to increase, so on hospital day four, the patient was taken to the operating room, found to have an ischemic cecum and descending colon, and received a total colectomy. Gross pathology revealed extensive pseudomembranes or raised yellow-white plaques overlying an erythematous and edematous mucosa. Microscopic evaluation demonstrated an inflammatory exudate composed of mucinous fibrinous material containing polymorphonuclear cells.

Discussion

This is an inflammatory condition of the colon caused by ingestion of the spore-forming anaerobic gram-positive bacillus, *Clostridium difficile*. The colonic inflammatory response is a result of toxin-induced cytokines (toxins A and B), and disease can range from mild diarrhea to life-threatening conditions such as toxic megacolon, perforation, or sepsis. Only strains of toxin producing *C. diff* cause disease and the pathopneumonic condition associated with CDI is pseudomembranous colitis. Recently, CDI has been associated with increased mortality. This has been attributed to an emerging strain of *C. diff* that has a mutation of the toxin regulatory gene *tcd* C. This strain (referred to as BI/NAP1/027) produces several-fold more toxin A and B as well as a binary toxin resulting in more severe disease.

Clostridium difficile is a ubiquitous organism found in soil and the environment; however, its major reservoir is within the hospital. Spores of *C. diff* have been recovered from hospital surfaces such as toilets, commodes, bedpans, floors, and thermometers. Spores can survive on surfaces for months and typical hospital cleaning products have no activity against them. It is the most common cause of acute care hospital-acquired diarrhea, accounting for 15% to 30% of all cases of antibiotic-associated diarrhea. No healthcare-acquired CDI benchmarks exist, but experts believe that 0.5% or fewer of all hospital admissions or discharges (or 10 CDIs per 10,000 patient-days, based on a length of stay of 5 days) is a reasonable target rate (D. Gerding, Hines Veterans Affairs Hospital, Chicago, personal communication); however, over the last 8 years, an increased incidence of CDI has been reported with rates in excess of 20 cases per 1,000 admissions and rates per 10,000 patient-days exceeding the target goal by more than ten-fold.

A number of clinical features have been described for CDI including malaise, anorexia, abdominal cramping, diarrhea, and fever. Systemic findings, such as fever and leukocytosis, are usually absent in mild disease but are common in moderate or severe disease. Renal failure and shock have also been described. Many facilities employ scoring criteria to determine severity. Several conditions, such as older age (>60), WBC greater than 15,000 or bandemia greater than 10%, elevated serum creatinine (≥1.5 times baseline), low albumin, and altered mental status may be markers for severe or complicated disease.

Objective evidence of colitis includes fever, cramps, leukocytosis, presence of leukocytes in feces, and colonic inflammation visualized by endoscopy or CT scan (colonic-wall thickening). Severe disease may cause paralytic ileus or toxic megacolon resulting in no diarrhea. Definitive diagnosis requires laboratory identification of *C. diff* toxin in a stool sample and/or visualization of pseudomembranes during endoscopy. Several methods are available to aid in the diagnosis of CDI, each with described advantages and disadvantages (Table 5.1).

Historically, metronidazole and oral vancomycin have been viewed as equivalent with regard to efficacy and relapse rates and thus, given the higher cost of oral vancomycin and the concern for the development of vancomycin-resistant enterococci, metronidazole, administered orally or intravenously, has typically

Table 5.1 Stool Tests for Diagnosis of *Clostridium Difficile* Infection[a]

Test	Detects	Advantages	Disadvantages
Cell cytotoxin assay	Primarily Toxin B	Standard; high sensitivity	Requires tissue culture facility; labor intense; takes 24–48 hours
Toxin enzyme immunoassay (EIA)	Toxin A or A and B	Fast (2–6 hours); easy to perform; high specificity	Not as sensitive as the cytotoxin assay
Glutamate dehydrogenase (GDH) enzyme immunoassay	*C. difficile* common antigen (GDH)	Fast (<1 hour); easy to perform; high negative predictive value	Must be combined with another method that detects toxin to verify diagnosis.
Culture	Toxigenic and nontoxigenic *C. difficile*	Permits strain typing in epidemics	Labor intense requiring anaerobic culture; cannot distinguish between toxin-producing strains; takes 2–5 days
Batched Real-time (RT) Polymerase Chain Reaction (PCR)	*tcdB* (toxin)	High sensitivity and specificity	Labor intense; typically run in daily batches; expensive
On demand Real-time (RT) Polymerase Chain Reaction (PCR)	*tcdB*, (toxin) *tcdC* deletion, and Binary Toxin (outbreak strain)	Rapid (<1 hour); high sensitivity and specificity	expensive

[a] Specimen should be watery, loose, or unformed and promptly submitted to the hospital laboratory.

been the preferred initial agent of choice. Vancomycin has been reserved for patients with severe disease, intolerance to metronidazole, those who failed to respond to metronidazole, or cases in which metronidazole is contraindicated (i.e., pregnancy). However, recent observational studies have suggested that metronidazole may have been associated with increased failure and recurrence rates when compared with treatment periods prior to the year 2000, and prospective trials have reported vancomycin to be superior to metronidazole in the setting of severe disease. In patients who are unable to tolerate oral medications, intracolonic vancomycin could be used (Table 5.2).

Management of Severe CDI

In patients with severe CDI, metronidazole should be given in combination with oral vancomycin. In the absence of ileus, metronidazole should be administered orally. With ileus, vancomycin should be administered via nasogastric tube or via rectal instillation. Although recommended for severe CDI, data have not demonstrated a difference in outcome when higher dosage regimens

Table 5.2 Treatment for *Clostridium Difficile* Infection

	Initial Episode		
	Mild to moderate disease	**Severe with normal bowel function**	**Severe with ileus**
Oral metronidazole 500 mg three times a day for 10 to14 days	X		
Oral vancomycin 125 mg enterally four times a day for 10 to14 days		X	
IV metronidazole 500 mg every 8 hours for 10 to14 days			X
Oral vancomycin 500 mg enterally four times a day for 10 to 14 days			X
Colectomy		May be required if no response to medical management	

Recurrence	
First	**Subsequent (≥2)**
Treatment with the same drug used to treat the first episode is recommended	Oral vancomycin 125 mg enterally four times a day for 10 to14 days followed by vancomycin taper or pulse dose over 4 to 6 weeks[a]
	Sequential oral vancomycin followed by rifaximin (resistance already described)
	Concomitant oral vancomycin with rifampin (resistance already described)
	Passive antibody
	Infuse donor stool

[a] Vancomycin rather than with metronidazole, in part because of the adverse effects (e.g., peripheral neuropathy) resulting from long-term exposure to metronidazole.

of vancomycin were used. Patients with possible severe CDI should undergo a surgical consultation as soon as possible, in the event that there is limited response to medical treatment. Clinical presentation suggestive of a poor outcome includes ileus, marked leukocytosis (>20,000 per μL), serum lactate greater than 5 mmol/L, and rising serum creatinine. Colectomy can be a life-saving procedure. Intravenous immunoglobulin use has been considered but outcomes have been mixed.

Management of Recurrent Clostridium difficile Infection

About 20% of patients with CDI will experience at least 1 additional episode and 45% of patients with one recurrence will have another, some with multiple relapses. Antibiotic resistance does not appear to be an issue in recurrent CDI. A first recurrence can be treated in the same manner as a first episode according to disease severity; however, metronidazole should not be utilized beyond treatment of the first recurrence and for durations exceeding 14 days because of the potential for toxicity, including both hepatotoxicity and polyneuropathy. For further recurrences, tapered or pulse dosing of vancomycin has been the most widely used regimen (see Table 5.2).

Adjunctive treatment with various therapies has been trialed. Probiotics, such as *Saccharomyces boulardii* or *Lactobacillus* GG have been used with hopes of repopulating the colonic microflora, and restricting the growth of toxigenic *C. diff*. Most studies are limited to a small number of patients. Saccharomyces has been associated with a beneficial effect on recurrence rates when added to and continued after treatment with metronidazole or vancomycin. Probiotics are generally safe and easy to administer in most patient populations; however, most studies have failed to demonstrate a consistent benefit of probiotics for the prevention of CDI.

There have been anecdotal reports of treatment success measured by resolution of symptoms with the use of oral vancomycin in combination with rifampin for patients with multiple relapses and a newer rifamycin, rifaximin, with poor GI absorption may have a potential role for treatment in this setting. Of note, however, wide-spread rifampin resistance has already been reported among *C. diff* isolates. Nitazoxanide, a nitrothiazolide compound, and fidaxomicin, a macrolide antibiotic, both have activity against *C. diff* and have been compared to oral vancomycin with similar efficacy results.

One last alternative therapy for recurrent CDI is fecal transplantation in hopes of restoring bacterial homeostasis. The donor specimen must be fresh and homogenized using normal saline. After filtration, the preparation is delivered by nasogastric tube. This treatment has been associated with a 94% cure rate (no recurrence) in survivors.

Control Measures

Environmental Contamination

As stated above, environmental surface contamination with *C. diff* spores is common, with the heaviest contamination on floors and carpets. Other sources of contamination include nurses' uniforms and other clothing, blood pressure cuffs, thermometers, telephones, call buttons, scales, and feeding tube equipment. Importantly, both asymptomatic patients (carriers) and patients with active disease contribute to this environmental contamination. Environmental cleaning and enhanced disinfection measures are needed. Although a variety of cleaning agents are effective in killing vegetative forms of *C. diff*, only chlorine-based disinfectants, high-concentration, vaporized hydrogen peroxide, or activated liquid hydrogen peroxide are sporicidal. Environmental cleaning with bleach solutions decrease surface contamination and this has been associated with a significant reduction in CDI.

Hand Contamination

Contamination of the hands of healthcare workers can lead to and result from contamination of the environment and it is well known that compliance with hand washing is not ideal. Additionally, alcohol-based hand rubs now commonly used for hand hygiene do not kill spores and are not effective at removing them from hands. Of note, it has been reported that *C. diff* contaminated hands could transfer, on average, 36% of spores after use of alcohol gels followed by handshaking. Hand washing (30 seconds to 2 minutes with soap and water) followed by proper hand drying with a disposable paper towel is effective for spore removal.

Patient Contamination

Previously, investigators reported that about two-thirds of patients colonized with *C. diff* become asymptomatic carriers and that asymptomatic carriage has been associated with lower levels of environmental contamination; however, recent data found that patients with documented CDI or asymptomatic carriage had high rates of skin contamination (61%–78%) and even noncarriers had skin contamination rates of 19%. Spores on the skin of patients are easily transferred to the hands of care providers. Cleansing patients with chlorhexidine-saturated cloths has been shown to reduce contamination of patient's skin and subsequently contamination of healthcare workers' hands.

Other Infection Control Measures

Barrier precautions (gloves and gown) and dedicated equipment have been recommended for any patient and or environmental contact. Various infection control measures including single-use rectal thermometers, endoscope disinfection, and limiting use of select antibiotics have also been described in guidelines. The use of a comprehensive bundle consisting of education, increased early case finding methodologies, expanded infection control measures, a *C. diff* management team, and targeted antimicrobial management has been associated with rapid and sustainable control.

Case Conclusion

Despite efforts, the patient remained severely hypotensive on multiple vasopressors, experienced ventricular fibrillation arrest, and expired 2 days after surgery.

Suggested Reading

Bartlett JG, Gerding DN. Clinical recognition and diagnosis of clostridium difficile infection. Clin Infect Dis 2008;46:S12–S18

Cohen S et al. Clinical practice guidelines for clostridium difficile infection in adults: 2010 update by the Society for Healthcare Epidemiology of America (SHEA) and the Infectious Diseases Society of America (IDSA). Infect Control Hosp Epidemiol 2010;31(5).

Loo VG et al. A predominantly clonal multi-institutional outbreak of clostridium difficile-associated diarrhea with high morbidity and mortality. NEJM 2005;353(23):2442–2449.

McFarland LV. Alternative treatments for Clostridium difficile disease: what really works? J Med Microbiol 2005;54(2):101–111.

Musher D et al. Relatively poor outcome after treatment of Clostridium difficile colitis with metronidazole. Clin Infect Dis 2005;40:1586–1590.

Muto CA et al. Control of an outbreak of infection with the hypervirulent clostridium difficile BI strain in a university hospital using a comprehensive "bundle" approach. Clin Infect Dis 2007;45(10):1266–1273.

Sunenshine RH and M. LC, Clostridium difficile-associated disease: new challenges from an established pathogen. Cleve Clin J Med 2006;73:187–197.

Zar FA et al. A comparison of vancomycin and metronidazole for the treatment of Clostridium difficile-associated diarrhea, stratified by disease severity. Clin Infect Dis 2007;45:302–307.

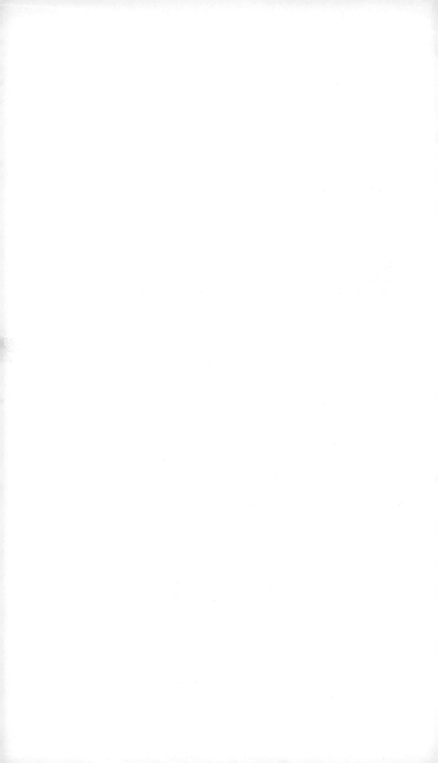

Chapter 5b

Herpes Simplex Virus Esophagitis

Andrew T. Root and Teresa R. Zembower

Initial Case Presentation

An 84-year-old woman with a history of chronic lymphocytic leukemia (CLL) (treated with rituximab 3 years ago and alemtuzumab 1 year ago) and chronic hepatitis B infection presents to the emergency department with a 2-week history of dysphagia, odynophagia, malaise, poor oral intake, and 5-pound weight loss. She is noted to be afebrile and mildly tachycardic with dry mucous membranes but an otherwise unremarkable oropharynx. Her chest is clear to auscultation and her cardiac and abdominal exams are otherwise normal. Routine laboratory studies reveal normal electrolytes, mild prerenal azotemia, and normal liver function tests as well as elevation in peripheral white blood cell count consistent with known CLL. Chest radiograph is unremarkable. Computed tomography of the chest, abdomen, and pelvis demonstrates marked wall thickening at the gastroesophageal junction.

The physician in the emergency department elects to admit the patient for intravenous (IV) hydration and further evaluation. The Gastroenterology Service is consulted and performs an upper endoscopy before an inpatient bed has even been assigned. Findings include multiple large, superficial ulcerations with normal intervening squamous mucosa (Fig. 5.1). Biopsies are taken, at which time the esophageal mucosa is noted to bleed quite easily. Therapy with a proton pump inhibitor and analgesics is initiated.

Differential Diagnosis and Initial Management

The possible etiology of esophagitis encompasses a wide range of infectious and noninfectious diseases. Noninfectious etiologies include gastroesophageal reflux disease, pill esophagitis, and malignancy, including adenocarcinoma, lymphoma, and Kaposi's sarcoma. The most common infectious causes of esophagitis are herpes simplex virus (HSV), cytomegalovirus, and Candida species. Less commonly, other viral (human immunodefiency virus (HIV), Epstein-Barr virus, varicella zoster virus, human papilloma virus) and fungal (*Cryptococcus neoformans, Histoplasma capsulatum, Blastomyces dermatiditis, Aspergillus* species) agents are implicated. Rarely, *Mycobacterium* species and *Nocardia* species[1] may

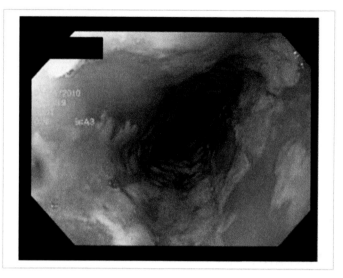

Figure 5.1 Upper endoscopy demonstrates multiple, large, superficial ulcerations with normal intervening squamous mucosa.

be implicated. Idiopathic aphthous ulcers have been identified in patients with acquired immunodefiency syndrome.[2]

Herpes simplex virus esophagitis (HSVE) most commonly represents reactivation of latent viral infection, with or without a specific history of symptomatic antecedent infection. However, primary infection of the esophagus may occur.[2] The majority of upper digestive herpetic infections are caused by HSV-1.[3]

Herpes simplex virus esophagitis is a common complication of immunosuppression and is most notably seen in patients who have undergone stem cell and solid organ transplantation as well as those with hematologic malignancies.[4] HSVE occurs less commonly in patients with HIV infection.[5] Other populations at risk include those treated with chemo- and radiotherapy, corticosteroids, and other immunosuppressive agents as well as patients with diabetes mellitus, alcoholism, and chronic cardiovascular and kidney disease.[2] Recent upper endoscopy or insertion of nasogastric tube have been reported in a high percentage of cases of HSVE, suggesting a possible role for trauma and/or viral autoinoculation in precipitating active disease.[2] Occurrence of HSVE in seemingly immunocompetent adults has been described, but remains rare and typically results in self-limited infection.[6]

The most common clinical manifestations of HSVE are dysphagia, odynophagia, and chest pain. Other less common symptoms are fever, nausea, vomiting, extraesophageal herpetic lesions, and gastrointestinal bleeding.[3] Patients may be asymptomatic. Rarely reported manifestations include tracheoesophageal fistula, food impaction, intractable hiccups, and esophageal perforation.[7–10]

Upper GI tract endoscopy is essential to the diagnosis of HSVE. Barium esophagography may be employed, in which case the nonspecific finding of small ulcerations in the distal esophagus would be typical. A large spectrum of endoscopic findings may be observed. Classically, findings predominantly involve the lower third of the esophagus.[3] Vesicles are seen early in the course. Often by the time endoscopy has been performed the vesicles have coalesced to form shallow, well-circumscribed, "volcano-like" ulcers, usually with normal-appearing intervening mucosa. Exudates, plaques, or diffuse erosions may also be seen.[4]

Brushings and biopsies should be taken from the edge of ulcers. Viral cytopathic effects include ground-glass nuclei with chromatin margination and multinucleated giant cells (Figs. 5.2 and 5.3). Histopathology may reveal Cowdry type A (eosinophilic nuclear) inclusions. Immunohistochemical stains may be helpful when other studies are inconclusive. Viral tissue culture is the most sensitive and specific test and allows for antiviral susceptibility testing, should it be clinically indicated.

Case Presentation (continued)

Pathology results reveal acute esophagitis with ulcerations as well as viral cytopathic effect (multinucleation, molding of nuclei and chromatin margination) consistent with HSV infection. Immunohistochemical stains are positive for HSV. Viral tissue cultures are pending. The patient's tachycardia and azotemia resolve but she continues to experience dysphagia and odynophagia with reduced oral intake. IV acyclovir is initiated.

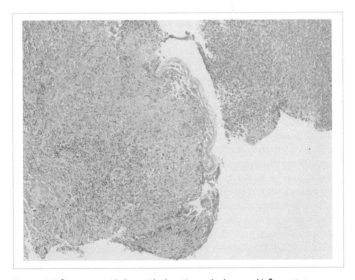

Figure 5.2 Squamous epithelium with ulceration and submucosal inflammatory exudate.

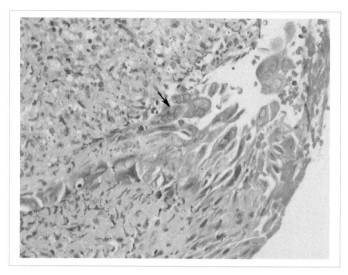

Figure 5.3 Higher magnification view with *arrow* identifying cell with multinucleation, molding of nuclei, and chromatin margination.

Management and Discussion

General management of esophagitis includes use of analgesics, and IV hydration and alimentation when clinically indicated. The condition may be self-limited, particularly in immunocompetent patients, but treatment is indicated to hasten recovery, limit dissemination, and prevent local complications such as bleeding or perforation. Acyclovir is the treatment of choice. Oral therapy (200–400 mg orally 3 to 5 times a day) is sufficient for those able to swallow pills, but IV administration (5 mg/kg IV every 8 hours) may be necessary for patients with severe odynophagia. Dosing should be adjusted based on renal function. When IV therapy is initiated, this can be transitioned to oral therapy to complete the treatment course after symptoms improve. There is limited experience with famciclovir and valacyclovir but these are acceptable alternatives, offering the advantage of decreased pill burden but the potential disadvantage of increased cost. Immunocompromised hosts should be treated for 14 to 21 days. In immunocompetent patients for whom symptoms are not yet improving at the time of diagnosis, a 7 to 10 day course is generally sufficient.

For patients who fail to respond to therapy with acyclovir in the first 5 to 7 days, drug resistance should be considered. This is often related to repeated exposure to acyclovir in the past, though HSV resistance has been reported in treatment-naïve patients.[11] Ongoing infection is unlikely in immunocompetent patients, in whom the disease is generally self-limited.[6] Foscarnet is the drug of choice for resistant HSV strains, though it is associated with significant toxicity and requires IV administration.

Primary prophylactic acyclovir can be considered in high-risk patients, and indeed may already be part of a post-transplantation antimicrobial regimen for many individuals. Patients with advanced HIV infection are unlikely to benefit from primary prophylaxis. For those patients with severe or frequent recurrences, a secondary prophylactic or suppressive regimen (acyclovir 600–1,000 mg daily in 3–5 divided doses) can be administered.

Case Conclusion

The patient's dysphagia and odynophagia improve significantly over the next 48 hours such that she is able to eat and drink comfortably. Viral tissue cultures are positive for HSV-1. She is transitioned to oral valacyclovir and discharged home. Three weeks later she finishes a course of therapy with complete resolution of her symptoms. Eight months later she experiences a relapse of HSVE, presenting with similar symptoms and is again treated successfully with acyclovir.

References

Sutton FM, Graham DY, Goodgame RW. Infectious esophagitis. Gastrointest Endosc Clin N Am 1994;4:713.

Généreau T, Rozenberg F, Bouchaud O, Marche C, Lortholary O. Herpes esophagitis: a comprehensive review. Clin Microbiol Infect 1997;4:397–407.

Généreau T, Lortholary O, Bouchaud O, et al. Herpes simplex esophagitis in patients with AIDS: Report of 34 cases. Clin Infect Dis 1996;22:926–931.

McBane RD, Gross Jr JB. Herpes esophagitis: clinical syndrome, endoscopic appearance, and diagnosis in 23 patients. Gastrointest Endosc 1991;37(6):600–603.

Bini EJ, Micale PL, Weinshel EH. Natural history of HIV-associated esophageal disease in the era of protease inhibitor therapy. Dig Dis Sci 2000;45:1301.

Ramanathan J, Rammouni M, Baran Jr J, Khatib R. Herpes simplex esophagitis in the immunocompetent host: an overview. Am J Gastroenterol 2000;95:2171–2176.

Cirillo NW, Lyon DT, Schuller AM. Tracheoesophageal fistula complicating herpes esophagitis in AIDS. Am J Gastroenterol 1993;88:587–589.

Marshall JB, Smart JR 3rd, Elmer C, et al. Herpes esophagitis causing an unsuspected esophageal food bolus impaction in an institutionalized patient. J Clin Gastroenterol 1992;15:179.

Mulhall BP, Nelson B, Rogers L, Wong RK. Herpetic esophagitis and intractable hiccups (singultus) in an immunocompetent patient. Gastrointest Endosc 2003;57:796.

Cronstedt JL, Bouchama A, Hainau B, Halim M, Khouqeer F, Al Darsouny T. Spontaneous esophageal perforation in herpes simplex esophagitis. Am J Gastroenterol 1992;87:124–127.

Kriesel JD, Spruance SL, Prichard M, et al. Recurrent antiviral-resistant genital herpes in an immunocompetent patient. J Infect Dis 2005;192:156.

Acknowledgement

The authors would like to thank Ikuo Hirano, Chao Qi, and Xianzhong Ding for their assistance with the included figures.

Chapter 5c

Norovirus in the Healthcare Setting

Sarah Miller and Sara Cosgrove

Initial Case Presentation

A 32-year-old otherwise healthy registered nurse who works on the transplant surgery unit presents to the emergency room with complaints of nausea, vomiting, and diarrhea for 2 days. She reports that she was working the day shift yesterday when she suddenly felt nauseous and vomited in the staff bathroom. She subsequently left work early. Overnight, she had several more episodes of nonbloody emesis, as well as watery diarrhea. She denies abdominal pain. After an episode of presyncope, she asked her husband to bring her to the emergency room for IV fluid hydration.

On evaluation, she is noted to have a fever of 38.4°C. Her blood pressure while supine is 82/50 mmHg and she is orthostatic. Her exam is otherwise remarkable only for dry mucous membranes. The abdominal exam is benign. She continues to have watery diarrhea and despite IV fluid resuscitation remains orthostatic and lightheaded. She is therefore admitted to the medical floor for further observation and IV fluids. She reports to the admitting intern that she had cared for a renal transplant patient with similar symptoms on her unit the day before the onset of her symptoms. The patient denies any other sick contacts. She also denies any new or unusual foods. She and her husband ate the same food for dinner the night before and for breakfast the day of the onset of symptoms, and he has not had any similar symptoms. She has no recent travel history.

Differential Diagnosis and Initial Management

Acute gastroenteritis is a common entity and is a major cause of serious morbidity and death globally among adults and children. In most cases, the causative agent is not specifically identified. Recent technology has allowed for recognition of an increasing number of cases caused by viruses, specifically rotavirus and norovirus. Rotavirus is the main agent of acute gastroenteritis among infants and young children, with a peak incidence in the winter months. Bacterial agents can cause the syndrome either by producing toxins that are subsequently ingested or by direct infection. *Staphylococcus aureus* and *Bacillus cereus* both produce toxins that, once ingested, cause nausea, vomiting, and diarrhea usually within 6 hours. *Clostridium perfringens* produces toxin after spores germinate, usually 12 to 24 hours after ingestion. Other bacterial pathogens such as *E. coli*, *Vibrio*, *Salmonella*, *Shigella*, *Yersinia*, and *Campylobacter* can cause gastroenteritis in which diarrhea tends to be a more prominent component of the syndrome and generally have a longer incubation period of more than 24 hours. Parasitic causes of gastroenteritis include *Cryptosporidium*, *Giardia*, and *Entamoeba*. Several features of the history may suggest the most likely etiologic agents, such as the presence of blood or mucus in the stool, associated fever, recent ingestion of certain foods, antibiotic use, travel history, and immune status. In the setting of a gastroenteritis outbreak, one should consider certain pathogens, including *S. aureus*, *Bacillus cereus*, *C. perfringens*, *E. coli*, *Salmonella*, *Shigella*, *Campylobacter*, *Vibrio*, rotavirus, and noroviruses.[1]

This case highlights the typical epidemiology and clinical features of acute gastroenteritis caused by norovirus. Noroviruses were first identified as a cause of gastrointestinal illness in 1972 from stool samples collected during an outbreak in Norwalk, Ohio in 1968.[2] They are a group of nonenveloped, single-stranded RNA viruses. The noroviruses include at least four serotypes: the Norwalk, Hawaii, Snow Mountain, and Taunton viruses.[1] They are the major etiologic agents of acute nonbacterial gastroenteritis and the most common cause of epidemic gastroenteritis. It is estimated that the noroviruses are responsible for more than 50% of gastroenteritis outbreaks worldwide.[1] They have been linked to outbreaks in such environments as hospitals, nursing homes, schools, dormitories, prisons, camps, daycare centers, military posts, restaurants, and cruise ships.[1–3,5,9,15] Outbreaks occur throughout the year but peak during cold weather months. The noroviruses are estimated to cause 21 million illnesses, 50,000 hospitalizations, and 310 deaths in the United States annually.[3]

The noroviruses are highly contagious; the infectious dose is as low as 10 to 100 virions.[4] Transmission can occur with person to-person contact, consumption of contaminated food or water, and via contact with contaminated environmental surfaces.[1,5] Information compiled from several investigations suggests that norovirus outbreaks primarily involve person-to-person transmission. Transmission most often occurs through the fecal-oral route. However, noroviruses have also been detected in vomitus and transmission via aerosolized vomitus has been reported.[1] Viral shedding can begin during the prodrome phase of illness, and peaks at 2 to 5 days after inoculation. At the peak, there are approximately 100 billion viral copies per gram of feces.[5] Detection of the virus in stool persists for an average of 4 weeks following infection. Viral shedding may persist for several weeks or months in immunocompromised patients. Up to 30% of norovirus infections are asymptomatic.[6] The amount of viral shedding among asymptomatic patients is likely less than that from symptomatic patients, but may be sufficient to transmit infection.

The incubation period ranges from 10 to 51 hours, with an average incubation period of 24 to 36 hours. The illness is usually mild and typically lasts an average of 24 to 72 hours.[1,3] However, symptoms can last as long as 4 to 6 days in certain patient populations, including children, the elderly, and immunocompromised persons.[7] The clinical syndrome typically includes acute onset of diarrhea, nausea, vomiting, anorexia, and abdominal discomfort. The stools are characteristically loose, watery, and nonbloody. Patients may also experience low-grade fever (in about one-third to half of cases), chills, headache, and myalgias.

A clinical diagnosis of norovirus may be made in the setting of an outbreak in the absence of another documented pathogen, but it is difficult to make a definitive diagnosis based solely on the signs and symptoms, as they are non-specific. Several advances have been made in the laboratory diagnosis of norovirus. Clinical laboratories in hospitals rarely routinely test for norovirus and diagnostics are often restricted to outbreak investigations. Some clinical laboratories perform real-time reverse transcription PCR (RT-PCR) assays on stool specimens. These assays have not been cleared by the FDA but commercial kits are available.[5] The sensitivity of the RT-PCR depends on the primers used, and it is challenging to develop a comprehensive set of primers given the genetic diversity of noroviruses. The RIDASCREEN is an FDA-approved enzyme immunoassay (EIA) for detection of norovirus antigens in stool, which has been used for preliminary detection of norovirus during outbreaks. The sensitivity of EIA ranges from 36% to 80%, and specificity ranges from 47% to 100%.[5] The CDC recommends that negative EIA results be confirmed by RT-PCR during an outbreak.[5] The noroviruses do not grow in cell culture.

Case Presentation (continued)

Several stool studies are sent, including stool culture and *C. difficile* assay, and return negative. Overnight, she is able to tolerate a clear liquid diet. The patient's symptoms resolve with supportive care in approximately 24 hours, and she is discharged from the hospital. That evening, she receives a call from her unit's manager, asking if she can work the day shift the following day. They are currently short-staffed because several nurses and other staff members are ill with the same GI illness. The patient feels well, and agrees to work the next day.

Discussion and Management

There currently is no specific therapy for norovirus gastroenteritis, and treatment consists of supportive measures. Regardless of the underlying cause of gastroenteritis, hydration with oral and IV fluids is the mainstay of treatment and should be started even before pursuing diagnostics.[1] Oral rehydration solution (ORS) is commercially available and can be prepared according to a specific formula. ORS is typically adequate to replace fluid losses, but if uncontrolled vomiting or severe dehydration occur, replacement with isotonic IV fluids may be necessary. Antimotility agents such as loperamide may provide some benefit, but have not been formally studied in the management of norovirus-associated diarrhea.[6] Bismuth subsalicylate has been shown to reduce the duration of gastrointestinal symptoms among patients with norovirus, but had no effect on the volume of stool passed or viral shedding.[8] Other supportive treatment measures include administration of antiemetics and analgesics for symptom management.

Another important aspect of norovirus management involves implementation of infection control measures to prevent or control an outbreak, particularly in healthcare facilities. The general approach to prevention and control of norovirus infections includes proper hand hygiene, decontamination of surfaces and materials, and avoidance of person-to-person contact. Johnston and colleagues describe an outbreak in a large urban hospital, in which termination of the outbreak required temporary closure of affected units, decontamination of the environment, screening of patients and healthcare workers, and furlough of ill healthcare workers.[9] The CDC published updated guidelines on norovirus outbreak management and disease prevention in March 2011 (Table 5.3).[5]

Appropriate hand hygiene is likely the single most effective measure to prevent transmission of norovirus. Handwashing with soap and water will remove viral particles from the hands, although the duration of handwashing must be prolonged. In one study, 60 seconds of handwashing with soap and water, followed by rinsing for 20 seconds and drying with a disposable towel completely removed norovirus from hands.[10] The efficacy of alcohol-based and other hand sanitizers has not been established. A study comparing the effectiveness of water rinse only, antibacterial soap, and alcohol-based hand sanitizer at various concentrations for norovirus elimination from the hands found that alcohol-based hand sanitizer at varying concentrations was the least effective intervention.[11] Another study of norovirus outbreaks in long-term care facilities found that facilities reporting that staff were equally or more likely to use alcohol-based hand sanitizers rather than hand washing had higher odds of an outbreak than facilities with staff less likely to use alcohol-based hand sanitizers.[12] Based on this information, handwashing with soap and water is recommended during norovirus outbreaks.

Noroviruses can withstand harsh conditions to survive on surfaces and objects. They can survive freezing and heat up to 140°F. They are also stable in chlorinated water (up to a concentration of 6.25 mg/L), and are acid resistant and ether stable. Norovirus has been detected on surfaces such as computer keyboards, soap dispensers, blood pressure cuffs, pulse oximeters, tympanic thermometers, furniture, and toilets.[13] The use of chemical disinfectants to

Table 5.3 Key Points Regarding Investigation and Management of a Norovirus Outbreak
• Initiate investigations promptly.
• Attempt to identify predominant mode of transmission and possible source.
• Promote good hand hygiene, preferably with soap and water
• Exclude ill staff for a minimum of 48 hours, preferably 72 hours. This includes food handlers, patient-care workers, childcare providers.
• After cleaning surfaces to remove soiling, disinfect using 1,000–5,000 ppm (1:50–1:10 dilution) of household bleach or other EPA-approved disinfectant.
• Collect whole stool specimens from at least 5 persons during acute phase of illness for diagnosis by PCR or EIA. Negative EIA should be confirmed by PCR.
• Report all outbreaks to state and local health departments.
Adapted from CDC. Updated norovirus outbreak management and diseases prevention guidelines. MMWR 2011;60:1–15.

decontaminate environmental surfaces is an important component of infection control during a norovirus outbreak, as fomites have been found to be sources of infection in outbreaks. The efficacy of chlorine beach (sodium hypochlorite) is well established. The CDC recommends use of a chlorine bleach solution at a concentration of 1,000 to 5,000 ppm on hard, nonporous surfaces.[5] This approach has been found to be superior to cleaning with quaternary ammonium compounds, detergents, and alcohol for feline caliciviruses.[5,6,9,10] Heat disinfection with temperatures higher than 140°F is recommended for items that cannot be disinfected with a bleach solution.

Given the highly contagious nature of norovirus, isolation of symptomatic persons can be a very effective means of halting transmission and propagation of an outbreak. The underlying principle is to minimize person-to-person contact during the peak period of viral shedding, which includes the period of clinical illness and the first 24 to 72 hours of the recovery phase. The CDC recommends contact precautions with isolation gowns and gloves in outbreak settings and when there is risk of contamination with infected vomitus or feces. Although there are no recommendations regarding wearing of masks, some may argue for their use, particularly in the presence of actively vomiting persons given the risk of transmission through aerosolized vomitus. In some situations, exclusion of exposed and potentially incubating persons is necessary. In the hospital setting, identification of a norovirus outbreak often results in ward closures. Ill patients may be housed together on a single unit or cohorted in rooms with a dedicated nursing staff. Patients with proven or suspected norovirus infection should not be transferred to other units or facilities, if this can be avoided.

In addition to the strategies described above for control of patient-to-patient transmission, patient contact by ill healthcare workers should be avoided. The CDC recommends that workers who have worked in potentially affected areas not be transferred to or work on unaffected areas for 48 hours after exposure to reduce spread by incubating or asymptomatically infected individuals.[5] Ill staff members and food handlers should be instructed to remain off of work during their illness and for 48 to 72 hours following resolution of symptoms. In a study comparing exclusion of affected staff for 48 versus 72 hours in nursing homes, there was found to be a lower overall attack rate among staff in the 72-hour exclusion group, but no significant difference in the mean number of cases, attack rate among the nursing home residents, or in the duration of outbreaks.[14] Some suggest that food handlers should be restricted from handling ready-to-eat food or kitchenware for an additional 72 hours after returning to work.[15]

Case Conclusion

When the patient arrived at work the following morning, she found that access to the unit was blocked off and several staff members were standing outside in the hall. She was informed that about one-third of the patients on the unit had developed GI symptoms and several tested positive for norovirus. All of the affected patients had been transferred to another unit overnight. She was asked some screening questions by an infection control practitioner, and was asked to go home and return when she had been free of symptoms for 72 hours. The transplant unit was thoroughly disinfected with bleach over the course of the day, and new patients were admitted after the cleaning process was completed. None of the newly admitted patients developed a similar diarrheal illness.

References

Mandell GL, Bennett JE, Dolin R. Mandell, Douglas, and Bennett's principles and practice of infectious diseases, 7th ed. Philadelphia: Churchill Livingston, 2009.

Kapikian AZ, Wyatt RG, Dolin R, Thornhill TS, Kalica AR, Chanock RM. Visualization by immune electron microscopy of a 27-nm particle associated with acute infectious nonbacterial gastroenteritis. J Virol 1972;10:1075–1081.

Goldman L, Ausiello D. Cecil Medicine, 23rd ed. Philadelphia: Saunders, 2007.

Zingg W, Colombo C, Jucker T, Bossart W, Ruef C. Impact of an outbreak of norovirus infection on hospital resources. Infect Control Hosp Epidemiol 2005;25:263–267.

Centers for Disease Control and Prevention. Updated norovirus outbreak management and diseases prevention guidelines. MMWR 2011;60:1–15.

Koo HL, Ajami N, Atmar RL, DuPont HL. Noroviruses: the leading cause of gastroenteritis worldwide. Discov Med 2010;10:61–70.

Goodgame R. Norovirus gastroenteritis. Curr Infect Dis Rep 2007;9:102–109.

Steinhoff MC, Douglas RG Jr, Greenberg HB, Callahan DR. Bismuth subsalicylate therapy of viral gastroenteritis. Gastroenterology 1980;78:1495–1499.

Johnston CP, Qiu H, Ticehurst JR, et al. Outbreak management and implications of a nosocomial norovirus outbreak. Clin Infect Dis 2007;45:534–540.

Barker J, Vipond IB, Bloomfield SF. Effects of cleaning and disinfection in reducing the spread of norovirus contamination via environmental surfaces. J Hosp Infect 2004;58:42–49.

Liu P, Yuen Y, Hsiao HM, Jaykus LA, Moe C. Effectiveness of liquid soap and hand sanitizer against Norwalk virus on contaminated hands. Appl Environ Microbiol 2010;76:394–399.

Blaney DD, Daly ER, Kirkland KB, Tongren JE, Kelso PT, Talbot EA. Use of alcohol-based hand sanitizers as a risk factor for norovirus outbreaks in long-term care facilities in northern New England: December 2006 to March 2007. Am J Infect Control 2011;39:296–301.

Morter S, Bennet G, Fish J, et al. Norovirus in the hospital setting: virus introduction and spread within the hospital environment. J Hosp Infect 2011;77:106–112.

Vivancos R, Sundkvist T, Barker D, Burton J, Nair P. Effect of exclusion policy on the control of outbreaks of suspected viral gastroenteritis: Analysis of outbreak investigations in care homes. Am J Infect Control 2010;38:139–143.

Centers for Disease Control and Prevention. Norovirus outbreak associated with ill food-service workers—Michigan, January-February 2006. MMWR 2007;56:1212–1216.

Chapter 5d

Postoperative Intraabdominal Infection

David S. Yassa and Sharon B. Wright

Initial Case Presentation

A 33-year-old female with a history of Roux-en Y gastric bypass 7 years prior complicated by anastomotic leak has since experienced chronic abdominal pain, recurrent obstructions and undergone repeated abdominal procedures for lysis of adhesions. Most recently, she underwent exploratory laparotomy with adhesiolysis and placement of mesh for abdominal closure 5 months prior to admission. Two weeks prior to admission, she was seen in a local emergency department and admitted briefly for intravenous antibiotics and discharged on a 10-day course of cephalexin for treatment of abdominal cellulitis.

On the day of admission, the patient was seen for a complaint of abdominal pain. On the initial examination, she was noted to have a temperature of 38.5°C, diffuse abdominal tenderness with rebound and guarding throughout, as well as diminished bowel sounds. Her abdominal incision was well-healed without surrounding erythema or drainage. Her white blood cell count was 14,500/ul with a marked neutrophil predominance. She was ultimately admitted to the hospital for further evaluation and management.

Differential Diagnosis and Initial Management

The differential diagnosis to consider for the patient's abdominal pain, fever, and leukocytosis is broad in this case. Independent of her prior abdominal procedures and subsequent complications, multiple other etiologies would have to be considered. Acute cholecystitis, appendicitis, pancreatitis, diverticular disease, urinary tract infection, and pelvic inflammatory disease with or without tuboovarian abscess could all manifest with these signs and symptoms. Additionally, her history of multiple previous abdominal procedures and bowel obstructions requiring surgery for lysis of adhesions raises the possibility of recurrent small bowel obstruction.

Given that the patient had implantation of a mesh foreign body to facilitate abdominal closure 5 months previously, surgical site infection must be considered as a likely possibility. The mesh may act as a "privileged" or sequestered site, perpetually infected for months or even years prior to manifestation of signs and symptoms. In contrast to infections occurring in the absence of implanted material, for the purposes of surveillance, infections such as the one described in this case are considered surgical site infections for up to 1 year following the implantation of prostheses and foreign material. This distinction is made based on criteria set forth by the National Healthcare Safety Network, a voluntary reporting and surveillance system established by the CDC Division of Healthcare Quality Promotion. Further complicating matters, perforated abdominal viscous with or without abscess formation must remain high on the differential diagnosis, due both to the prior history of anastomotic breakdown and the grave consequences of missing such a diagnosis.

In the case of abdominal pain with fever, particularly when bowel perforation is suspected, immediate laboratory evaluation and imaging of the abdomen is important (though not absolutely necessary) before operative intervention. When labs are obtained, marked leukocytosis may be noted, although this is a fairly nonspecific finding. Abnormalities in liver function tests may be suggestive of biliary involvement. When assessing for possible pancreatitis, an elevated serum lipase level may be slightly more specific for pancreatic pathology than an abnormal amylase.

In some cases of abdominal pain and fever after surgery, a clinical history, physical examination and upright chest radiograph demonstrating intraperitoneal free air may be sufficient to make the diagnosis of perforated bowel. However, a negative x-ray does not exclude the diagnosis. Plain abdominal radiographs are typically much less sensitive than the chest x-ray for detecting free air. In the majority of cases, cross sectional imaging (such as with computed tomography) is especially useful. If there is evidence of associated systemic inflammatory response syndrome (SIRS) or sepsis in a patient with abdominal pain and fever after surgery, routine blood cultures should be obtained to rule out concurrent bacteremia.

Case Presentation (continued)

Computed tomography (CT) scanning of the abdomen revealed free fluid, a large duodenal diverticulum, and possible perforation with likely retroperitoneal abscess. The patient was resuscitated with IV fluids and vancomycin and piperacillin-tazobactam were prescribed to cover for likely pathogens originating in the gut lumen (including methicillin-resistant strains of *Staphylococcus aureus* in light of the prior contact with the healthcare system). The patient was urgently rushed to the operating room for emergent exploratory laparotomy with repair of a perforated duodenal ulcer, drainage of a large retroperitoneal abscess, gastrostomy with gastric drainage catheter insertion, and placement of drains. Postoperatively, the patient was maintained on therapy with vancomycin and piperacillin-tazobactam. Unfortunately, over the first several hours after surgery, the patient experienced high spiking fever and ultimately developed hypotension and other signs consistent with postoperative SIRS/sepsis. She was returned to the OR for repeat exploratory laparotomy about 18 hours after the initial procedure. Over the ensuing 48 hours, she developed right flank pain and erythema and was found to have likely fasciitis related to spread of her infectious process through her retroperitoneum as seen on her CT scan. On postoperative day 7, she underwent further drainage and debridement of the right retroperitoneum and abdominal wall via a right flank incision.

Management and Discussion

As was noted, the patient presented with an acute abdominal process in the context of extensive prior surgical instrumentation and recent exposure to the healthcare setting. She underwent CT scanning that further defined the extent of the infection. The patient was appropriately started on broad-spectrum antimicrobial therapy with agents active against both community- and healthcare-associated intraabdominal infection as soon as the diagnosis of intraabdominal infection with associated SIRS was suspected. This case demonstrates the need for prompt institution of effective antimicrobial therapy in cases of suspected intraabdominal infection as well as the need for urgent or even emergent operative intervention directed at source control of the infection.

Source control, which includes the elimination of infectious foci through operative management, percutaneous drainage, and attempts to restore anatomical function, is imperative and should occur in most cases with minimal delay. Percutaneous drainage of abscesses or other collections may be preferable for well-contained infections and are recommended whenever possible.[1] Extensive infection, the presence of peritonitis, persistent or enlarging collections in spite of percutaneous drainage attempts, ongoing clinical instability, and grossly abnormal anatomy, as was evident in this case, are all factors that would favor open surgical intervention. Several factors are known to predict failure of source control including severe illness, poor nutritional status, extensive peritoneal involvement, presence of malignancy, and failure of initial attempts at debridement.[1] For this reason, maintaining adequate nutritional status during the perioperative period (through enteral or parenteral nutrition if bowel rest is deemed necessary,) is an important measure to aid in the prevention of complicated postoperative abdominal infection.

Culture of deep space, infected material may assist in guiding therapy in the case of a high risk or healthcare-associated infection. The organisms associated with complicated intraabdominal infections include aerobic coliforms including *E. coli*, *Klebsiella* species, *Proteus mirablis* and *Enterobacter* species; anaerobic organisms including *Bacteroides* species (predominantly *Bacteroides fragilis*) and *Clostridial* species; and gram-positive aerobic cocci including *Streptococcus* species and enterococci.[1] An epidemiological shift towards more antimicrobial-resistant organisms including *Pseudomonas aeruginosa*, extended spectrum β-lactamase-producing gram-negative bacteria, and vancomycin-resistant enterococci (VRE) as well as *Candida* species may be observed in healthcare-associated infections. Empiric antimicrobial therapy should be chosen to cover the appropriate organisms based on local antimicrobial susceptibility data, which is outside of the scope of this review. While Gram stain alone may not contribute useful information in the case of a community-acquired infection, the presence of yeast noted on Gram stain from a healthcare-associated infection may be useful at least in making the decision to start empiric antifungal therapy.

Healthcare-associated intraabdominal infections require aggressive empirical antimicrobial therapy. A typical regimen will include multidrug therapy to ensure that resistant gram-negative organisms are covered. The decision to initiate empiric antifungal therapy prior to receipt of culture data may be based on results from Gram stain and in certain cases may be impacted by the immune status of the patient, presence of malignancy or findings of perforated viscus. Ultimately, the decision for continued therapy with a triazole or echinocandin should be guided by antifungal susceptibility testing. Empiric anti-*enterococcal* therapy based on local susceptibility data should be included in patients with immunocompromising conditions, cardiac valvular disease or intravascular devices. Therapy directed at VRE should be included in the initial empiric regimen for patients at high risk for such infections including liver transplant patients with a hepatobiliary source and patients known to be colonized with VRE.[1] Empiric coverage for obligate anaerobic organisms, particularly *Bacteroides fragilis* should be instituted, particularly if there is anatomic disruption of the small bowel, or colon.[1] In all cases, as culture data become available, therapy should be narrowed to address the identified pathogens.

Therapy for intraabdominal infections should continue for approximately 7 days after complete source control of the infection has been achieved and the patient shows signs of clinical improvement. It is less clear what the duration of therapy should be for patients with percutaneous drains in place. Different clinicians vary the length of therapy based on persistence or resolution of collections based on repeat radiographic imaging, drain output and clinical status. Some clinicians favor continuing antibiotics until all drains have been removed and others extend therapy for a period beyond the removal of all drains—neither of which has been definitively demonstrated as superior in the literature.

Intraabdominal infections in the postoperative patient remain a significant cause of morbidity and mortality. The Surgical Care Improvement Project (SCIP) is a program originally supported by the Center for Medicare and Medicaid Services aimed at the reduction and prevention of complications related to surgery overall, including the prevention of surgical site infection through adherence to best practice measures including antimicrobial prophylaxis selection, dosing, and timing of administration. The SCIP measures directed at prevention of postoperative infection, including many directed at the prevention of abdominal postoperative infection, are summarized in Table 5.4.[2]

As has already been noted, aggressive measures at source control, cultures in the case of healthcare-associated infection, optimization of nutritional status, and judicious use of antimicrobial therapy with tailoring based on susceptibility data may be particularly effective in preventing the development of infection with antimicrobial resistant organisms.

Case Conclusion

The patient remained in the hospital for a total of 80 days on antimicrobial therapy and total parenteral nutrition and underwent repeated retroperitoneal washout procedures and vacuum-assisted closure dressing changes for recurrent fever and abscesses. Ultimately, she was found to have additional

Table 5.4 **Strategies Endorsed by the Surgical Care Improvement Project in Support of the Prevention of Surgical Site Infections**
Prophylactic antibiotic received within 1 hour prior to surgical incision
Appropriate prophylactic antibiotic selection for surgical procedure
Prophylactic antibiotics discontinued within 24 hours after end of surgery (48 hours for cardiac procedures)
6 a.m. serum glucose <200 mg/dl in patients undergoing cardiac procedures on postoperative days 1 and 2
Appropriate hair removal for surgical patients
Postoperative normothermia for patients undergoing colorectal procedures
Urinary catheter removal on postoperative day 1 or 2
Perioperative temperature management to maintain normothermia

anterior intraabdominal abscess cavities that were managed with drains placed by an interventional radiologist. Cultures taken at the time of her repeated debridement and drainage procedures revealed the growth of VRE, *Candida albicans*, and *Stenotrophomonas maltophilia*. At the time of discharge, the patient was improved with healing abdominal and right flank wounds and no further fevers.

References

Solomkin JS, Mazuski JE, Bradley JS, et al. Diagnosis and management of complicated intra-abdominal infection in adults and children: guidelines by the Surgical Infection Society and the Infectious Diseases Society of America. Clin Infect Dis 2010;50(2):133–164.

Bratzler DW, Hunt DR. The surgical infection prevention and surgical care improvement projects: national initiatives to improve outcomes for patients having surgery. Clin Infect Dis 2006;43(3):322–330.

Suggested Reading

Laterre PF. Progress in medical management of intra-abdominal infection. Curr Opin Infect Dis 2008;21(4):393–398.

Solomkin JS, Mazuski J. Intra-abdominal Sepsis: Newer Interventional and Antimicrobial Therapies. Infect Dis Clin North Am 2009;23(3):593–608.

Solomkin JS, Mazuski JE, Bradley JS, et al. Diagnosis and management of complicated intra-abdominal infection in adults and children: guidelines by the Surgical Infection Society and the Infectious Diseases Society of America. Clin Infect Dis 2010;50(2):133–164.

Chapter 6a

Catheter-Associated Urinary Tract Infection

Courtney Hebert and Ari Robicsek

Initial Case Presentation

During her usual surveillance, an infection preventionist (IP) noted an increase in catheter associated urinary tract infections (CA-UTI) on the oncology unit of the local hospital. In just one week there appeared to be two new cases of CA-UTI, as well as an additional patient who came to her attention because of a multidrug-resistant organism (MDRO) isolated from the urine.

Patient A was a 35-year-old female with breast cancer who was hospitalized for pneumonia and required intensive care unit (ICU) admission. During a short stay in the intensive care unit a urinary catheter was placed. On hospital day 5 she developed a new fever and back pain and a urine culture was sent. On hospital day 6 the culture grew more than 100,000 cfu/ml *E. coli*. Prior to the fever she had been doing well, able to work with physical therapy and had been ambulating down the hall of the medical-surgical ward, holding her catheter bag, without difficulty.

Patient B was a 45-year-old police officer with a history of paraplegia secondary to a gunshot wound 10 years prior. He was admitted for treatment of head and neck cancer. At home he used intermittent bladder catheterization but had an indwelling catheter placed in the emergency room at the time of this admission. On day 10 of hospitalization he developed low grade fever and leukocytosis, and a urine culture grew more than 100,000 cfu/ml *Pseudomonas aeruginosa*.

The final case, patient C, has just come to the IP's attention today. She is an elderly woman with metastatic breast cancer who was hospitalized for pain control. She had previously been at a long term care facility (LTCF) and presented with an indwelling catheter which was left in place after hospital admission. On day 10 of her hospitalization she developed a gastrointestinal bleed and was sent to the ICU. She was afebrile and has no other sign of infection. A urine culture was sent and was positive for more than 100,000 cfu/ml *E. coli*. The microbiology lab reported that this isolate was resistant to fluoroquinolones, all cephalosporins and piperacillin-tazobactam.

Differential Diagnosis and Initial Management

Up to one quarter of hospitalized adult patients have an indwelling urinary catheter at some point during their hospital stay. Indwelling urinary catheters increase the risk of bladder infection by providing easy access from the environment to the normally sterile urinary tract. While a catheter is in place, the incidence of developing bacteriuria is 3% to 8% per day. Not surprisingly then, catheter-associated bacterial infection of the urinary tract is the most common healthcare-associated infection encountered in U.S. hospitals. Bacteriuria places patients at risk for upper urinary tract and bloodstream infection, and is a frequent reservoir for the emergence and proliferation of MDRO. These infections are estimated to cost the health care system over 500 million dollars each year in the United States.

Defining CA-UTI is not straightforward and definitions vary throughout the literature and guidelines. The CDC's National Health Safety Network (NHSN) definitions are summarized in Table 6.1. The most recent guidelines from the Infectious Disease Society of America use the following definition: Catheter associated bacteriuria is divided into CA-UTI and catheter associated asymptomatic bacteriuria (CA-ASB). Defining CA-UTI requires a urine culture positive for at least one organism ($\geq$100,000 cfu/ml) in a patient with an indwelling urinary catheter, or with a catheter that has been removed within the past 48 hours, and the patient *has signs or symptoms of UTI* with no other identifiable cause. In contrast, the definition of CA-ASB requires a urine culture with at least one organism ($\geq$100,000 cfu/ml) in a patient *without* symptoms of UTI. The NHSN guidelines have removed asymptomatic bacteriuria as an infection type.

Patient A met the criteria for CA-UTI and required treatment. As is common in hospitalized patients, she did not have a clear and sensible indication for catheterization. Appropriate indications for indwelling catheters include: (1) urinary retention that is not relived by medical or surgical routes; (2) incontinence if other methods fail or for comfort in a terminally ill patient; (3) patients who need strict urine output monitoring (such as patients with sepsis or other critical illness); and (4) perioperative need (in the operating room or postoperatively for select surgeries). Indwelling catheter use in patients without an appropriate indication needlessly exposes them to the risk of infection and should be avoided.

Patient B also fits into the definition of CA-UTI. He has a history of paraplegia and a neurogenic bladder. This is a population that is typically plagued with recurrent urinary infections because of their ongoing need for some form of catheterization. Alternatives to a chronic indwelling catheter for these patients include intermittent catheterization or suprapubic catheterization. Intermittent catheterization has been shown to decrease the risk of infection and should be the first choice whenever possible.

Patient C has CA-ASB. This is a common finding in LTCF patients who are catheterized. When she was transferred to the ICU for a noninfectious cause, a urine culture was inappropriately sent (Table 6.2). Guidelines recommend against screening for CA-ASB except in pregnant catheterized patients. This case also highlights a significant problem in infection control, namely that patients who have long-term indwelling catheters can become reservoirs for

Table 6.1 Updated NHSN criteria for Symptomatic Urinary Tract Infection

		Must Meet at Least 1 of the Following Criteria			
1a	**1b**	**2a**	**2b**	**3**	**4**
Patient has IUC[a] AND **At least one sign or symptom**[b] AND **Positive urine culture with ≥10⁵ CFU/ml**[c]	Patient does not have IUC AND At least one sign or symptom[d] AND Positive urine culture with ≥10⁵CFU[c]	Patient has IUC AND At least one sign or symptom[b] AND Positive urine culture with ≥10³ and <10⁵ CFU/ml[c] AND Positive urinalysis[e]	Patient does not have IUC AND At least one sign or symptom[d] AND Positive urine culture with ≥10³ and <10⁵ CFU/ml[c] AND Positive urinalysis[e]	Patient ≤1 year of age with or without IUC AND At least one sign or symptom[f] AND Positive urine culture with ≥10⁵ CFU/ml[c]	Patient ≤1 year of age with or without IUC AND At least one sign or symptom[f] AND Positive urine culture with ≥10³ and <10⁵ CFU/ml[c] AND Positive urinalysis[e]
OR		**OR**			
Patient had IUC removed within last 48 hours AND **At least one sign or symptom**[b] AND **Positive urine culture with >10⁵ CFU**[c]		Patient had IUC removed within last 48 hours AND At least one sign or symptom[b] AND Positive urine culture with ≥10³ and <10⁵ CFU/ml[c] AND Positive urinalysis[e]			

[a] IUC, indwelling urinary catheter.

[b] Signs or symptoms include temperature >38°C, suprapubic tenderness or costovertebral angle pain or tenderness (with no other recognized cause for these symptoms).

[c] With no more than 2 species present in culture.

[d] Signs or symptoms include temperature >38 C in a patient who is ≤65 years of age, urgency, frequency, dysuria, suprapubic tenderness, or costovertebral angle pain or tenderness (with no other recognized cause for these symptoms).

[e] Positive urinalysis is defined as one of the following: (1) positive dipstick for leukocyte esterase and/or nitrite, (2) pyuria (urine specimen with ≥10 WBC/mm³ of unspun urine or ≥3 WBC/high powered field of spun urine), (3) microorganisms seen on Gram stain of unspun urine.

[f] Signs or symptoms for infants include temperature >38°C (core), <36°C (core), apnea, bradycardia, dysuria, lethargy, or vomiting.

Table 6.2 **Appropriate and Inappropriate Use of Urine Culture**	
Appropriate Use of Urine Culture	**Inappropriate Use of Urine Culture**
Patients with symptoms of urinary infections such as:	On admission for screening purposes
	When a catheter is removed
Pain with urination	Test of urinary tract infection cure (after treatment)
Frequency of urination	
Fever or rigors	Malodorous or cloudy urine without symptoms
Flank pain	
New change in mental status without another cause	Routine surveillance

highly resistant bacteria. This is especially common at LTCF. When these patients are admitted to acute care hospitals they can expose other hospitalized patients to MDRO.

Case Presentation (Continued)

Patient A's catheter was removed immediately without any complications and she was treated with ciprofloxacin with gradual improvement in her symptoms. She was ultimately discharged home to finish a 14 day course of oral ciprofloxacin.

Patient B developed high fevers despite the initiation of therapy with ciprofloxacin and was subsequently found to have positive blood cultures for *Pseudomonas aeruginosa* resistant to fluoroquinolones. The infectious disease consultant recommended removing his central venous catheter when his blood cultures remained positive for a second day. He also insisted that his urinary catheter be removed. The antibiotic was then changed to piperacillin-tazobactam because no oral antibiotics would cover this isolate. His insurance plan did not cover home intravenous antibiotics so he remained in the hospital for an additional 14 days solely for antibiotic treatment. At the end of this treatment he had a new central venous catheter placed for future chemotherapy and he was discharged home. His indwelling urinary catheter was removed without complications and his doctors recommended that he return to intermittent catheterization.

Patient C was initially started on cefepime when her urine culture turned positive. When the susceptibility testing returned and the isolate was found to be resistant to many antibiotics, she was switched to meropenem and contact isolation was implemented. Her gastrointestinal bleed resolved and she was discharged to the general ward four days later where she finished a 14 day course of meropenem. A urine culture sent a few days after finishing treatment grew *E. coli* resistant to meropenem as well as more than 100,000 cfu/ml of *Candida albicans*. This time her doctors decided not to treat her with antibiotics. A few weeks later, the IP noticed that there had been an increase in highly resistant *E. coli* in the ICU and an outbreak investigation was started.

Two cases of CA-UTI on the same ward within a week was concerning, but could potentially be a coincidence rather than a true increase in incidence. To investigate further the IP looked back over the past year and found that in the past 3 months the incidence of CA-UTI had tripled compared to the 9 previous months. After talking to some of the nursing managers and resident physicians she realized that there has been a lack of education about proper indications for indwelling urinary catheters and no recent initiative to try to decrease the use of these devices. While observing several catheter insertions she further noted deviations from sterile procedure and later found a patient in the hallway with his catheter bag on his lap in a wheelchair.

Acting on behalf of the hospital's infection control program, she decided to coordinate a series of lunchtime meetings to educate the nurses on this unit about proper insertion techniques and catheter maintenance. These recommendations included a reminder to keep catheter bags below the level of the bladder and a review of sterile technique. She also spoke to the internal medicine residency program about appropriate indications for catheter use and prompt removal when no longer needed. In addition she sent a memo to attending physicians reminding them of the indications for catheter use and removal. See Table 6.3, which summarizes the prevention strategies she recommended.

The hospital has an electronic health record, which she decided to use to her advantage. She first requested a report that showed catheter utilization by nursing units over time, and presented this to each nursing unit in turn in order to help limit inappropriate catheter use. Her final intervention was to schedule a meeting with the clinical decision support team. She planned to create an ongoing, electronic reminder to physicians to remove catheters when no longer needed.

Management and Discussion

Patient A and B were correctly diagnosed with CA-UTI and started immediately on appropriate treatment. Because Patient A showed signs of upper tract infection and Patient B was bacteremic they were both treated with a full 14-day course of antibiotics. Although not relevant to these two cases, the most

Table 6.3 Proper Use and Maintenance of Urinary Catheters

Prior to Catheter Placement	During Catheter Placement	After Catheter Placement
Make a formal hospital policy outlining appropriate indications for urinary catheters	Use aseptic technique when inserting catheter	Keep catheter bag below the level of the bladder
Educate nurses and physicians about appropriate indications for urinary catheters	Train staff in the appropriate way to insert catheter	Give individualized feedback on rates of CAUTI to wards
Require a physician's order to place a urinary catheter	Use a closed-catheter system	Create electronic reminders to remove catheters when no longer indicated

recent guidelines allow for shorter courses for patients with CA-UTI without complicating factors who respond quickly to antibiotics. In both cases A and B, the indwelling catheters were appropriately removed. Patient A's catheter was never indicated and Patient B will have a lower risk of infection with intermittent catheterization rather than chronic indwelling catheterization. Patient B's hospitalization was prolonged by many days and he required removal and reinsertion of a central venous catheter, all of which needlessly added to his healthcare exposure and costs.

Patient C's case illustrates a common practice in hospitalized patients with indwelling catheters. This patient did not have CA-UTI, but instead had CA-ASB. With or without the presence of a urinary catheter, CA-ASB has not generally been associated with poor outcomes among community-dwelling or hospitalized patients. In these cases treatment is not indicated and increases the risk that the patient could become colonized with more resistant bacteria. The most appropriate intervention the physicians should have made was simply to remove the indwelling catheter.

Patient C's second urine culture also grew *Candida albicans*. This is a common finding in urine cultures from patients with indwelling urinary catheters. Generally if the patient is asymptomatic, treatment is not indicated. If symptomatic, or in severely immunocompromised patients or patients who are undergoing urologic procedures, treatment may be considered. Avoiding inappropriate treatment for candiduria is yet another reason why urine cultures should only be sent when clinically indicated.

The IP's response to these cases was consistent with current guidelines, which recommend care provider education and catheter removal. Clearly preventing catheter insertion in the first place is the best way to avoid CA-UTI. When this is not possible, then the goal becomes prompt removal once the catheter is no longer indicated. Unfortunately it is common for healthcare providers to be unaware that their patients have indwelling catheters. Computer based reminders for nurses or physicians are effective at reducing catheter days. The IP's decision to try to use the capabilities of the EHR was both forward-thinking and in line with current recommendations.

Case Conclusion

These three cases illustrate the complexity of diagnosis, treatment and prevention of CA-UTI. These patients had their hospitalizations needlessly complicated by CA-UTI or in the case of Patient C, was unnecessarily exposed to antibiotic therapy. The IP's implementation of appropriate quality improvement measures will hopefully prevent these bad outcomes for future patients. All three patients have done well since hospital discharge.

Suggested Reading

Gould CV, Umscheid CA, Agarwal RK, Kuntz G, Peques DA, Healthcare Infection Control Practices Advisory Committee. Guideline for prevention of catheter-associated urinary tract infections 2009. Infect Control Hosp Epidemiol 2010;31(4):319–326.

Hooton TM, Bradley SF, Cardenas DD, Colgan R, Geerlings SE, Rice JC, et al. Diagnosis, prevention, and treatment of catheter-associated urinary tract infection in adults: 2009 international clinical practice guidelines from the Infectious Diseases Society of America. Clin Infect Dis 2010;50(5):625–663.

Horan TC, Andrus M, Dudeck MA. CDC/NHSN surveillance definition of health care-associated infection and criteria for specific types of infections in the acute care setting. Am J Infect Control 2008;36:309–332.

Trautner BW. Management of catheter-associated urinary tract infection (CAUTI). Curr Opin Infect Dis 2010;23(1):76–82.

Chapter 7a

Healthcare-Associated Infection after Solid Organ Transplant

Charlesnika T. Evans and Michael G. Ison

Case Presentation

The patient is a 48-year-old African American male who underwent cadaveric renal transplant 1 week prior to presentation. He has a history of hypertension, diabetes mellitus, coronary artery disease, hypercholesterolemia, and morbid obesity (BMI = 43). He is currently taking tacrolimus, mycophenolate mofitil, valganciclovir, trimethoprim-sulfamethoxazole, clotrimazole troches, insulin, aspirin, simvastatin, and metoprolol. Additionally, he received alemtuzumab and methylprednisolone for induction immunosuppression perioperatively. Clinically he did well after transplantation, rapidly made urine, and had a decline in his creatinine from 6.4 mg/dl immediately pretransplant to 2.2 on postoperative day 2. He returns now for routine postsurgical follow-up and is noted to have erythema, pain, and induration around the inferior one-third of the incision; he has had no fevers. No purulent drainage is expressed on palpation and his white blood cell count is 3.2; creatinine is 1.1 mg/dl. Two staples are removed from the incision and he is started on an oral first generation cephalosporin.

Differential Diagnosis and Initial Management

Solid-organ transplantation (SOT) is now considered the definitive management option for most patients with end-stage organ failure. Improvements in surgical techniques, immune suppression, and antimicrobial prophylaxis have reduced the frequency of rejection and prolonged graft survival after SOT. However, infections, whether they are healthcare-associated, opportunistic, or community-acquired remain a significant and frequent cause of morbidity and mortality following SOT. In general, infectious complications occur in three major time periods: early (0–30 days posttransplant), during peak immune suppression (31–180 days post-transplant), and late (181+ days posttransplant). Although healthcare-associated infections can occur at any time, most occur during the early posttransplant period and are typical of other healthcare-associated infections recognized after elective surgery. Presentation, though, is often modulated by the use of immune suppression; as a result, signs and symptoms may be muted.

The development of pneumonia, bloodstream infection (BSI), surgical site infection (SSI), and urinary tract infection (UTI) occur in all types of transplantation, although they vary by solid organ received. For example, there is a higher rate of pneumonia among lung transplant recipients and a higher rate of UTI among renal transplant recipients. Reported rates of pneumonia, BSI, and UTI episodes in heart and lung transplantation range from 14 to 138 infections per 100 patients for pneumonia, 4.1 to 29 infections per 100 patients for BSI, and 2.6 to 21.6 infections per 100 patients for UTI. Most HAIs occur within the first 30 days posttransplantation and SSIs are the most frequent within this time period, although post-transplant wound infections can occur up to a year after surgery. These infections are highest in abdominal transplantation (kidney and liver), with estimates from the literature up to 18.6% in kidney transplantation and up to 37.6% for liver transplantation. The Centers for Disease Control and Prevention (CDC) National Healthcare Safety Network (NHSN) collects data on HAIs in over 1,000 medical facilities; however, only 9 are transplant centers. The limited NHSN data suggest that SSIs in high-risk kidney transplant (6.6/100 operations) and liver transplant recipients (20.1/100 operations) are higher than in comparable nontransplant procedures (4.5 and 13.7, respectively). The most common risk factors for SSI have included patient demographic and medical characteristics such as age, body mass index, severe hyperglycemia, and surgery characteristics such as duration of operation and previous surgery.

Initial management of individual HAIs should be consistent with local standard-of-care practice and antimicrobial resistance patterns and detailed management guidelines are available from the American Society of Transplantation's Infectious Diseases Community of Practice. Some important points to note include: (1) Renal function is often abnormal in most transplant recipients; as such, any prescribed antimicrobial should be adjusted based on the individual patient's estimated creatinine clearance. (2) Drug interactions between frequently prescribed antimicrobials and antirejection medications complicate the management of such patients and may result in either over- or under-immunosuppression. (3) Foreign bodies (i.e., ureteral stents, biliary T-tubes) may be placed during the transplant procedure and should be taken into consideration in determining the duration of antimicrobial therapy. Discontinuation of antimicrobial therapy before removal of such foreign bodies may allow the infection to relapse. (4) Involvement of the transplant team (especially Transplant Infectious Diseases clinicians if available) at your center is critical. They may often be aware of unique surgical or host characteristics useful for diagnosis and management of the infection. (5) It is critical to consider the donor as the source of any early post-transplant infections presenting in the recipient. A careful review of all donor cultures should be conducted to help inform concern about a potential disease transmission. If a donor-derived disease transmission is considered, this should be reported immediately to the leadership at your transplant center, to your local organ procurement organization, and the national Organ Procurement and Transplant Network (currently the United Network for Organ Sharing). This is critical because it may avert morbidity and mortality in other recipients and is currently required by OPTN policy.

Case Presentation (continued)

The patient returned three days later with worsening erythema, pain, and induration despite being compliant with his antibiotic. He also noted low-grade temperature (to 100.5°F) at home and his peripheral WBC was 5.4. He was admitted and started on vancomycin and meropenem. CT imaging revealed a fluid collection deep to the wound and aspirated fluid grew an extended spectrum β-lactamase (ESBL) producing *Klebsiella pneumoniae*. Blood cultures remained negative.

Discussion and Management

Risk factors for infections with antibiotic-resistant microorganisms include comorbidities and underlying illness, hospitalization, invasive instrumentation (i.e., indwelling devices, mechanical ventilation), and previous antibiotic exposure. The latter, antibiotic exposure, has been associated with acquiring a variety of antibiotic-resistant microorganisms, such as methicillin-resistant *Staphylococcus aureus* (MRSA), vancomycin-resistant *enterococci* (VRE), and multidrug-resistant gram negatives. The prevalence of these resistant organisms varies by region and many of these organisms have been increasing in transplant recipients and can cause significant morbidity and mortality.

Methicillin-resistant *S. aureus* is responsible for 2.7% to 24% of SSIs in SOT recipients and 5.9% of BSIs. Colonization with MRSA in liver transplant recipients is associated with a high incidence rate of MRSA infection (31% to 87%). Reports have indicated that VRE may cause 5% to 11% of infections in liver recipients. Resistance in gram-negative organisms, such as ESBL-producing or carbapenem-resistant *Klebsiella* or *Pseudomonas,* are also increasing among SOT recipients. One study found that in SSIs, 80% of *K. pneumoniae* were ESBL-producing and 33.3% of *P. aeruginosa* isolates were carbapenem-resistant among kidney recipients.

Because both resistant pathogens and unusual infections (i.e., Mycobacteria, fungi) may be responsible for infections that fail to response to initial therapy, routine cultures of the affected organ system are critical and should be obtained whenever possible before antimicrobial therapy is instituted. Likewise, known colonization of the recipient with resistant pathogens (such as MRSA or VRE) may help guide initial therapy while cultures are still pending.

Prevention and Next Steps

Both the CDC and the American College of Surgeons, through the National Surgical Quality Improvement Program, have extensively studied and developed guidance to minimize post-surgical HAIs in nontransplant settings (Table 7.1).

Table 7.1 Summary of CDC Recommendations for Prevention of Surgical Site Infection

Recommendation	Level of Evidence for Recommendation[a]
Preoperative	
Preparation of the patient including: treating all current infections, hair removal, obtaining appropriate chemistry/hematology tests, and preoperative maintenance of surgical area	Category IA-IB, Category II
Hand/forearm antisepsis for surgical team members including cutting and cleaning nails and scrubbing arms	Category IB, Category II
Management of infected or colonized surgical personnel through education and encouragement of reporting of symptoms and developing policies related to personnel responsibility, work restrictions, and clearance to resume work	Category IB
Appropriate antimicrobial prophylaxis	Category IA-IB
Intraoperative	
Maintenance of appropriate ventilation in operating room	Category IB, Category II
Cleaning and disinfection of environmental surfaces	Category IB, Category II
Performance of environmental microbiologic sampling only in cases of epidemiologic investigation	Category IB
Appropriate sterilization of surgical instruments	Category IB
Use and changing of surgical attire (masks, gloves, gowns), when appropriate	Category IB
Adherence to aseptic technique	Category IA-IB, Category II
Postoperative incision care	
Protection of incision with sterile dressing and use of sterile technique and washing hands when changing dressings	Category IB, Category II
Education of patients and family about proper care of incision and potential symptoms of infection	Category II
Surveillance	
Use CDC definitions for SSI case finding; conducting both surveillance in the inpatient setting and postdischarge.	Category IB, Category II
Document surgical wound classification and variables known to be associated with SSI risk.	Category IB, Category II
Calculate and review SSI rates periodically.	Category IB

[a] *Category IA.* Strongly recommended for implementation and supported by well-designed experimental, clinical, or epidemiological studies. *Category IB.* Strongly recommended for implementation and supported by some experimental, clinical, or epidemiological studies and strong theoretical rationale. *Category II.* Suggested for implementation and supported by suggestive clinical or epidemiological studies or theoretical rationale.

Recommendations for prevention of SSI focus on preoperative patient and surgical team factors, intraoperative issues related to the environment of the operating room and aseptic technique, postoperative incision care, and conducting appropriate surveillance for SSIs in the inpatient setting as well as postdischarge. However, little work has been performed in transplantation. Additional work is needed to improve the current surveillance for HAI in SOT and develop interventions to reduce the rate of HAI.

Case Conclusion

After initial clinical improvement and appropriate drainage of the fluid collection, the patient's antibiotic regimen was reduced to meropenem and he received a total of 14 days and was discharged from the hospital. He was seen in follow-up 7 days later and had resolution of his infection. He continues to do well.

Suggested Reading

Edwards JR, Peterson KD, Mu Y, et al. National Healthcare Safety Network (NHSN) report: data summary for 2006 through 2008, issued December 2009. Am J Infect Control 2009;37:783–805.

Fishman JA. Infection in Solid-Organ Transplant Recipients. NEJM 2007;357:2601–2614.

Garzoni C and the AST Infectious Diseases Community of Practice. Multiply resistant gram-positive bacteria: Methicillin-resistant, vancomycin-intermediate and vancomycin-resistant Staphylococcus aureus (MRSA, VISA, VRSA) in solid organ transplant recipients. Am J Transplant 2009;9(Suppl 4):S41–49.

Hellinger WC, Crook JE, Heckman MG, et al. Surgical site infection after liver transplantation: Risk factors and association with graft loss or death. Transplantation 2009;87:1387–1393.

Ison MG, Hager J, Blumberg E, et al. Donor-derived disease transmission events in the United States: Data reviewed by the OPTN/UNOS Disease Transmission Advisory Committee. Am J Transplant. 2009;9:1929–1935.

Kidney Disease: Improving Global Outcomes (KDIGO) Transplant Work Group. KDIGO clinical practice guideline for the care of kidney transplant recipients. Am J Transplant. 2009;9 Suppl 3:S1–155.

Lynch RJ, Ranney DN, Shijie C, Lee DS, Samala N, Englesbe MJ. Obesity, surgical site infection, and outcome following renal transplantation. Ann Surg 2009;250:1014–1020.

Mangram AJ, Horan TC, Pearson ML, Silver LC, Jarvis WR, and the Hospital Infection Control Practices Advisory Committee. Guideline for prevention of surgical site infection. Infect Control Hosp Epidemiol 1999;20:247–278.

Mattner F, Fischer S, Weissbrodt H, et al. Post-operative nosocomial infections after lung and heart transplantation. J Heart Lung Transplant 2007;26:241–249.

Menezes FG, Wey SB, Peres CA, Medina-Pestana JO, Camargo LFA. Risk factors for surgical site infection in kidney transplant recipients. Infect Control Hosp Epidemiol 2008;29:771–773.

Munoz P and the AST Infectious Diseases Community of Practice. Multiply resistant gram-positive bacteria: Vancomycin-resistant enterococcus in solid organ transplant recipients. Am J Transplant 2009;9(Suppl 4):S50–56.

van Delden C, Blumberg EA, and the AST Infectious Diseases Community of Practice. Multidrug resistant gram-negative bacteria in solid organ transplant recipients. Am J Transplant 2009;9(Suppl 4):S27–34.

Chapter 7b

Hospital Acquired Infections in Hematopoietic Stem Cell Transplant Recipients

Nicole Theodoropoulos and Michael G. Ison

Case Presentation

A 45-year-old woman with acute myeloid leukemia was admitted for alloge-neic hematopoietic stem cell transplant (HSCT) with myeloablative condition-ing. Her absolute neutrophil count was low (100 cells/mm^3) on admission with an unknown duration of neutropenia. She was started on prophylactic cipro-floxacin, fluconazole, and acyclovir. On day +5 after HSCT, she had fevers to 102° F. The patient had no focal complaints. Exam was only notable for oral mucositis and a peripherally inserted central catheter (PICC) in the right arm that was intact and without tenderness or erythema at the insertion site. Pertinent laboratory results were an absolute neutrophil count of 0, normal chemistry and liver function panels, and a screening rectal swab positive for vancomycin-resistant enterococcus (VRE). Blood and urine cultures were sent and empiric antibiotics (cefepime) were started.

Differential Diagnosis and Initial Management

HSCT is often a curative measure for many malignancies, but carries a signifi-cant morbidity and mortality from infection, graft versus host disease (GVHD) and other medication related toxicities. Often, HSCT recipients are in the hos-pital for long periods of time (i.e., months) and are, therefore, at risk for many hospital acquired infections. The types of infection seen in HSCT recipients vary by the posttransplant phases (Figure 7.1). In the preengraftment phase (15–45 days depending on type of HSCT), severe neutropenia and breakdown of mucosal surfaces lead to increased risk of infection with bacteria (usually gas-trointestinal (GI) flora or gram positive organisms via central venous access), *Candida* species (from GI tract), and reactivation of Herpes Simplex virus (HSV). The postengraftment phase (from engraftment to day +100) is a time of weakened cellular and humoral immunity and acute GVHD. Therefore, infec-tions with *Aspergillus*, *Candida* and *Pneumocystis* are seen in addition to bacterial infections and reactivation of cytomegalovirus (CMV) and Epstein-Barr virus (EBV). The late phase after HSCT (>day +100) is a time when B cell and CD4+

T cell recovery is just beginning to occur and risk of infection is increased in patients being treated for chronic GVHD. The most common infections seen are those with encapsulated bacteria, *Aspergillus, Pneumocystis*, varicella zoster virus (VZV), CMV and EBV. Respiratory viral infections can be seen at any stage after HSCT and are often more severe than in immune competent patients.

The patient in our case is in the pre-engraftment period, but is noted to be at higher risk for opportunistic infection as she was neutropenic for an unknown period of time prior to admission. The differential diagnosis for the cause of this patient's febrile neutropenia includes line associated blood stream infection, candidemia or bacterial blood stream infection from gut translocation due to mucositis or aspergillosis (given prolonged neutropenia). Although the majority of patients like the one presented in our case will have fever during neutropenia, only 20% to 30% of them will have an infectious cause documented.

Any antipseudomonal β-lactam antibiotic (cefepime, piperacillin-tazobactam, imipenem or meropenem) is an appropriate initial empiric antibiotic in this situation. These antibiotics will have broad coverage against susceptible gram-positive and gram-negative organisms found in the mouth and throughout the GI tract that are likely to cause infection in this patient. If a patient has a serious allergy (i.e., immediate hypersensitivity or anaphylactic response) to penicillin or cephalosporins, therapy with a fluoroquinolone or aztreonam plus vancomycin would be a reasonable alternative option. Therapy against resistant organisms for which a patient is known to be colonized or from which the patient has been infected in the past should be added early, especially if the patient becomes hemodynamically unstable. For instance, we know our patient is colonized with VRE. Therefore, addition of daptomycin or linezolid should be

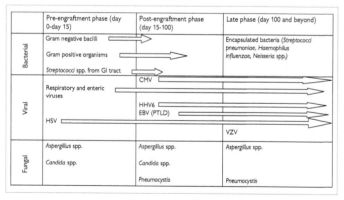

	Pre-engraftment phase (day 0–day 15)	Post-engraftment phase (day 15–100)	Late phase (day 100 and beyond)
Bacterial	Gram negative bacilli Gram positive organisms Streptococci spp. from GI tract		Encapsulated bacteria (*Streptococci pneumoniae, Haemophilus influenzae, Neisseria spp.*)
Viral	Respiratory and enteric viruses HSV	CMV HHV6 EBV (PTLD)	VZV
Fungal	*Aspergillus* spp. *Candida* spp.	*Aspergillus* spp. *Candida* spp. *Pneumocystis*	*Aspergillus* spp. *Pneumocystis*

Figure 7.1 Sequence of Most Common Opportunistic Infections in the Allogeneic HSCT Recipient Population
CMV, cytomegalovirus; EBV, Epstein Barr virus; HHV6, human herpes virus-6; HSV, herpes simplex virus; PTLD, posttrans plantlymphoproliferative disease; VZV, varicella zoster virus

(Adapted from Figure 2, page 1152;Tomblyn M, Chiller T, Einsele H, Gress R, Sepkowitz K, Storek J, et al. Guidelines for preventing infectious complications among hematopoietic cell transplantation recipients: a global perspective. Biol Blood Marrow Transplant 2009;15(10):1143–1238.)

considered if she remains febrile, becomes unstable or is found to have gram-positive organisms in culture.

During periods of neutropenia, a careful physical exam should be performed daily. If the patient remains neutropenic and febrile for more than 5 days, the differential diagnosis should be reevaluated. In this patient, a high suspicion for invasive fungal infection will remain. Although fluconazole is effective at preventing infections with *Candida* species, it lacks activity against *Aspergillus* or other invasive molds; breakthrough infections with these pathogens can occur. After 5 to 7 days of fever, imaging and additional laboratory studies are often undertaken to identify the source of the persistent fever.

Case Presentation (continued)

The patient remained persistently febrile and neutropenic despite cefepime and daptomycin was added after 48 hours of fever. Blood and urine cultures were negative and chest radiograph was unrevealing. The patient remained febrile and without localizing symptoms. On day +7, a CT scan of the chest, abdomen, and pelvis was performed to look for a focus of infection. Nodular infiltrates were seen diffusely in both lungs (Figure 7.2). Bronchoscopy was performed. Bronchoalveolar lavage (BAL) cultures revealed fungal hyphae (with eventual growth of *Aspergillus fumigatus*) and BAL *Aspergillus* galactomannan antigen enzyme immunoassay (EIA) was elevated. A diagnosis of probable invasive pulmonary aspergillosis was made. There was concern that this *Aspergillus* infection was hospital-acquired, as there was construction occurring on the ward the patient was staying.

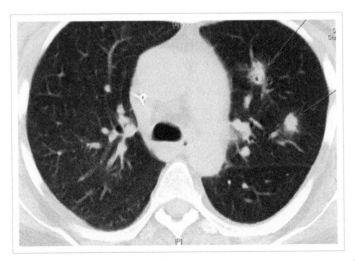

Figure 7.2 Computed Tomography (CT) Scan
Arrows show nodular infiltrates with surrounding ground glass opacity or "halo sign" which is consistent with invasive pulmonary aspergillosis.

Diagnosis, Management, and Prevention

Definite diagnosis of invasive pulmonary aspergillosis requires histopathological evidence of the fungus in the lung tissue, but probable diagnosis is made in this case by the combination of a high-risk patient with characteristic radiologic findings and a culture confirmation of *Aspergillus* species. The elevated galactomannan level in the BAL specimen is also very suggestive of aspergillosis, as galactomannan is a component of the *Aspergillus* cell wall. Serum galactomannan EIA is less sensitive than the test from BAL fluid and can also be falsely positive in the setting of piperacillin-tazobactam or amoxicillin-clavulanate use in addition to other fungal infections (histoplasmosis, blastomycosis or *Penicillium*).

Voriconazole is currently considered the preferred therapy for invasive disease due to *Aspergillus*. There is broad inter- and intrapatient variability in bioavailability of voriconazole, therefore therapeutic drug monitoring should be performed during treatment to ensure adequate serum levels of the drug. Optimal salvage therapy, in case of progressive disease despite initial therapy, is not established but lipid formulations of amphotericin B, caspofungin, micafungin, and posaconazole have been used alone or in different combinations with anecdotal success. Surgical resection is sometimes warranted. Obviously, the improvement of immune function is also paramount to successfully treating this disease.

Prevention of invasive aspergillosis in HSCT is an important and ever-evolving issue. Fluconazole has no antimold activity, but in a recent study comparing voriconazole to fluconazole prophylaxis in allogeneic HSCT patients, the fungal-free survival and overall survival was not improved with voriconazole. Posaconazole has been shown to be effective mold prophylaxis in high risk leukemia patients with GVHD.

Since *Aspergillus* is a pervasive mold that is found in soil, water, fruits, and vegetables, it is difficult to completely eradicate from the hospital. Increased numbers of *Aspergillus* spores in the air are often found during hospital construction. Although most *Aspergillus* transmission is airborne, hospital water supplies have also been implicated. Ways to prevent spread of aspergillosis in the hospital include high-efficiency particulate air (HEPA)-filter air purifiers, laminar airflow systems and asking patients to wear masks outside of their rooms. Increased actions to control mold should occur during times of construction. Water leaks should be promptly cleaned up and floors should be smooth and without carpet. Vacuum cleaning and other dust-producing cleaning mechanisms should be avoided in hospital wards for immunocompromised patients.

Case Conclusion

The patient was started on voriconazole. She engrafted on day +20 and neutrophil count returned to normal. Her fevers resolved. Voriconazole trough levels were monitored and in the therapeutic range (2–4 mg/L). She was discharged home in stable condition.

Suggested Reading

Ascioglu S, Rex JH, de Pauw B, et al. Defining opportunistic invasive fungal infections in immunocompromised patients with cancer and hematopoietic stem cell transplants: an international consensus. Clin Infect Dis 2002;34(1):7–14.

Freifeld AG, Bow EJ, Sepkowitz KA, et al. Clinical practice guideline for the use of antimicrobial agents in neutropenic patients with cancer: 2010 update by the infectious diseases society of america. Clin Infect Dis 2011;52(4):e56–93.

Krishna G, AbuTarif M, Xuan F, Martinho M, Angulo D, Cornely OA. Pharmacokinetics of oral posaconazole in neutropenic patients receiving chemotherapy for acute myelogenous leukemia or myelodysplastic syndrome. Pharmacotherapy 2008;28(10):1223–1232.

Marr KA. Fungal infections in oncology patients: update on epidemiology, prevention, and treatment. Curr Opin Oncol 2010;22(2):138–142.

Perlroth J, Choi B, Spellberg B. Nosocomial fungal infections: epidemiology, diagnosis, and treatment. Med Mycol 2007;45(4):321–346.

Salgado CD, Ison MG. Should clinicians worry about vancomycin-resistant Enterococcus bloodstream infections? Bone Marrow Transplant 2006;38(12):771–774.

Tomblyn M, Chiller T, Einsele H, et al. Guidelines for preventing infectious complications among hematopoietic cell transplantation recipients: a global perspective. Biol Blood Marrow Transplant 2009;15(10):1143–1238.

Trifilio S, Pennick G, Pi J, et al. Monitoring plasma voriconazole levels may be necessary to avoid subtherapeutic levels in hematopoietic stem cell transplant recipients. Cancer 2007;109(8):1532–1535.

Walsh TJ, Anaissie EJ, Denning DW, et al. Treatment of aspergillosis: clinical practice guidelines of the Infectious Diseases Society of America. Clin Infect Dis 2008;46(3):327–360.

Wingard JR, Carter SL, Walsh TJ, et al. Randomized, double-blind trial of fluconazole versus voriconazole for prevention of invasive fungal infection after allogeneic hematopoietic cell transplantation. Blood 2010;116(24):5111–5118.

Chapter 8a

Sepsis in a Very Low Birth Weight Neonate

Sandra Fowler

Case Presentation

Baby Girl A was born at 25 weeks gestation via spontaneous vaginal delivery. Birth weight was 980 grams. Maternal history was significant for incompetent cervix and group B strep bacteriuria. The infant was intubated minutes after delivery, and had placement of umbilical venous and arterial catheters. Blood cultures were obtained and the infant was started on ampicillin and gentamicin on admission to the neonatal intensive care unit (NICU). She required high-frequency jet ventilation by day 2 of life and was noted on routine screening to have skin colonization with methicillin-resistant *Staphylococcus aureus* (MRSA) on day 4. Umbilical catheters were discontinued after five days and a PICC was placed in the right basilic vein. Antibiotics were discontinued after 7 days. Though requiring intensive support, she was stable, and reached full oral feeds on day of life 19.

On day of life 22, she began having episodes of oxygen desaturation associated with increasing respiratory acidosis and abdominal distension. A sepsis workup was performed and the infant was started on vancomycin and piperacillin-tazobactam. Feeds were discontinued and nasogastric suction begun. Radiographs showed right upper lobe atelectasis and patchy infiltrates; ileus was also noted, but there was no free air or pneumatosis intestinalis. The endotracheal aspirate Gram stain showed numerous white blood cells, and few gram-positive cocci. Cultures of blood from the PICC, peripheral vein, and endotracheal aspirate were positive for MRSA. CSF and urine cultures remained negative.

Differential Diagnosis and Initial Management

This infant's clinical, imaging, and laboratory findings are consistent with nosocomial (late-onset) sepsis and pneumonia. Late-onset sepsis has generally been defined as sepsis that presents at greater than 48 to 72 hours of life. Infants being cared for in the NICU are at increased risk for nosocomial sepsis, particularly preterm infants and those with very low birth weight (VLBW). Nosocomial bloodstream infections complicate up to 20% of NICU hospitalizations for VLBW infants (<1500 grams) and this high susceptibility can be attributed to the immaturity of the neonatal immune system and skin, presence of indwelling catheters, prolonged hyperalimentation, prolonged mechanical ventilation, as well as surgical procedures such as central line placement and ligation of a patent ductus arteriosus. Among general NICU populations, the organisms responsible for nosocomial sepsis (Table 8.1) are predominantly gram-positive bacteria, many of which are multidrug-resistant, such as coagulase-negative staphylococci, MRSA, and vancomycin-resistant enterococci. However, gram-negative bacteria, including multidrug-resistant strains, may cause 15% to 30% of nosocomial sepsis in some institutions. *Candida* species has also been reported with increased frequency. This epidemiology should be considered when decisions regarding empiric therapy are made for the neonate presenting with suspected late-onset sepsis. Broad-spectrum antimicrobials are typically initiated with deescalation once the pathogen responsible for the infection has been identified. In one large multicenter survey, 70% of the episodes of sepsis in VLBW infants were caused by gram positive bacteria, of which 10% were due to *Staphylococcus aureus*. The proportion owing to MRSA varies, but is occurring with increasing frequency. The community-associated phenotype has emerged as the dominant MRSA strain causing healthcare-acquired infection in the NICU. Importantly, virulence factors associated with this USA300 clone are now appearing in methicillin-susceptible *Staphylococcus aureus* (MSSA) isolates, such that infection with either agent cannot be distinguished on clinical

Table 8.1 Distribution of Pathogens Associated with the First Episode of Late-Onset Sepsis: NICHD Neonatal Research Network

Organism	Number	Percentage
Gram-positive organisms	922	70.2
Staphylococcus (coagulase-negative)	629	47.9
Staphylococcus aureus	103	7.8
Enterococcus sp	43	3.3
Group B streptococcus	30	2.3
Other gram-positives	117	8.9
Gram-negative organisms	231	17.6
Escherichia coli	64	4.9
Klebsiella	52	4.0
Pseudomonas	35	2.7
Enterobacter	33	2.5
Serratia	29	2.2
Other gram-negative organisms	18	1.4
Fungi	160	12.2
Candida albicans	76	5.8
Candida parapsilosis	54	4.1
Other fungi	30	2.3
Total	1313	100

Used with permission from Carey AJ, Saiman L, Polin RA. Hospital-acquired infections in the NICU: Epidemiology for the new millennium. Clin Perinatol 2008;35:223–249.

grounds. Common signs of bloodstream infection are nonspecific and include temperature instability, apnea, hypoxia, and leukocytosis. Other typical sites of infection from MRSA include skin and soft tissue, bone, joints, and heart. Meningitis caused by MRSA or MSSA is not common; however, meningitis in the setting of late-onset sepsis is likely underreported.

Full term, well-born infants are not immune to MRSA, but are more likely to present with pustular skin eruptions rather than bacteremia and sepsis. Maternal vaginal MRSA colonization has been reported at a rate of approximately 3% and vertical transmission of identical MRSA isolates has been described. Additionally, studies have shown vertical transmission of MRSA through contaminated breast milk. Despite this, routine vaginal cultures for identification of MRSA colonization among pregnant women has not been recommended.

Preceding colonization can also predispose to invasive MRSA infection. There is some observational evidence that decolonization using intranasal mupirocin with or without chlorhexidine bathing may be effective in limiting outbreaks of MRSA infection in the NICU; however, no randomized trials of the effectiveness of decolonization therapy or its effect on MRSA infection have been conducted among this population. In one outbreak which was controlled with universal use of mupirocin for all neonates, lower eradication rates were observed among infants who were nasotracheally intubated or who were receiving nasal continuous positive airway pressure. Universal use of topical agents such as mupirocin for MRSA decolonization must be carefully monitored as resistance may develop.

Case Presentation (continued)

On day of life 24 the PICC was removed and the pipericillin-tazobactam was discontinued. She was treated with a 14-day course of vancomycin, with subsequent negative blood cultures. She gradually was returned to oral feeds and was able to be converted to conventional ventilation on day of life 30.

Management and Prevention of Nosocomial Sepsis in the NICU

Vancomycin remains the treatment of choice for MRSA bacteremia in the neonate. Initial dosing is based on birth weight and chronological age and should be tailored to achieve trough levels of 15 to 20 mcg/ml. Linezolid may be used under the guidance of a pediatric infectious diseases specialist when vancomycin therapy fails or is not tolerated. Clindamycin does not cross the blood-brain barrier and should generally be avoided in the premature newborn with MRSA bacteremia. Combination therapy with rifampin is sometimes advocated because of its activity in biofilms, though there are no clinical trials to support this practice. Devices such as central venous catheters should be removed as quickly as possible to prevent metastatic infection.

As detailed in our case presentation, risks for nosocomial sepsis include both intrinsic (e.g., extreme immaturity) as well as extrinsic (e.g., medical devices) factors. As such, strategies to prevent nosocomial sepsis have focused on better understanding these factors and exploring measures to reduce risk. Selected strategies have included attempts to improve the barrier function of neonatal skin, attempts to enhance the function of the GI tract, prevention of *Candida* colonization, improving care of central venous catheters, and improving hand hygiene among healthcare workers. The results of recent select studies of these strategies are included in Table 8.2. The following measures have been recommended to reduce the frequency of nosocomial infections, are effective, and are relatively inexpensive: (1) Cleanse hands with an alcohol-based emollient; (2) avoid scrubbing the skin with brushes or harsh soaps; (3) don sterile gowns and gloves when inserting central lines or during dressing changes; (4) adopt antimicrobial stewardship programs to promote appropriate use of antimicrobial agents; (5) avoid medications associated with an increased risk of infection whenever possible (systemic steroids); (6) minimize practices which bypass normal skin barriers (e.g., venipuncture and heel sticks); (7) minimize central venous catheter days; (8) encourage aggressive advancement of enteral feeds and the use of breast milk; (9) maximize space and staffing patterns; and (10) isolate or cohort infants harboring virulent or resistant pathogens.

Infants with MRSA infection or colonization should be cohorted and placed in contact isolation with use of gowns and gloves for contact with the patient

Table 8.2 Selected Strategies to Reduce Nosocomial Sepsis in NICU Patients

Risk Factor	Strategy	Conclusions
Intrinsic Risk Factors		
Reduced barrier function of skin	Topical emollients	Improved neonatal skin condition but increased risk of nosocomial sepsis.
Reduced barrier function of gastrointestinal tract epithelium	Early enteral feeds Probiotics containing anaerobic organisms	Enteral feeds have been started earlier among infants without nosocomial sepsis. Decreased risk of sepsis associated with use of some probiotics.
Extrinsic Risk Factors		
Colonization with *Candida* spp.	Prophylactic fluconazole	Reduced rate of fungemia. No reduction in all-cause mortality rate.
Central venous catheters	Quality improvement initiative for insertion and maintenance techniques	Reduced rate of catheter-associated bloodstream infections.
Staff hands as reservoirs for potential pathogens	Hand hygiene product: alcohol versus chlorhexidine soap	Improved staff skin condition. No difference in nosocomial sepsis.

Adapted by permission from Saiman L. Strategies for prevention of nosocomial sepsis in the neonatal intensive care unit. Curr Opin Pediatr 2006;18:101–106.

and the immediate environment of care. Many institutions have implemented routine screening for nasal colonization, though the sensitivity of this strategy to identify CA-MRSA may be improved by adding other sites such as the umbilicus and perineum to the screening protocol. Routine screening of healthcare workers is not recommended, but may be useful in an outbreak setting. Molecular and agar-based rapid screening tests for MRSA colonization are commercially available. In an outbreak setting, molecular analysis to assess the relatedness of MRSA isolates should be performed.

Case Conclusion

The infant was placed in contact isolation at the time the MRSA screen returned positive at day of life 4, and remained on contact precautions for the duration of hospitalization. Infants with MRSA infection or colonization were cohorted together in the unit. The unit continued to experience sporadic cases of MRSA colonization and infection, but no clonal outbreaks were observed.

Suggested Reading

Carey A, Long S. Staphylococcus aureus: a continuously evolving and formidable pathogen in the neonatal intensive care unit. Clin Perinatol 2010;37:535–546.

Carey A, Saiman L, Polin R. Hospital acquired infections in the NICU: epidemiology for the new millenium. Clin Perinatol 2008;35:223–249.

Gerber SI Jr, Scott MV, Price JS, Dworkin MS, Filippell MB, Rearick T, et al. Management of outbreaks of methicillin-resistant Staphylococcus aureus infection in the neonatal intensive care unit: a consensus statement. Infect Control Hosp Epidemiol 2006;27:139–145.

Milstone A, Budd A, Shepard J, et al. Role of decolonization in a comprehensive strategy to reduce methicillin-resistant Staphylococcus aureus infections in the neonatal intensive care unit: an observational cohort study. Infect Control Hosp Epidemiol 2010;31:558–560.

Saiman L. Strategies for prevention of nosocomial sepsis in the neonatal intensive care unit. Curr Opin Pediatr 2006;18:101–106.

Song X, Cheung S, Klontz K, Short B, Campos J, Singh N. A stepwise approach to control an outbreak and ongoing transmission of methicillin-resistant Staphylococcus aureus in a neonatal intensive care unit. Am J Infect Control 2010;38:607–611.

Chapter 8b

Bordetella pertussis in Healthcare

Terry C. Dixon

Case Presentation

A one-month-old infant born at 38 weeks gestation was seen in the pediatric emergency department for apnea. Physical exam was unremarkable except for increased nasal congestion with clear rhinorrhea. She was admitted for a diagnostic work-up consisting of a complete blood count with differential, serum electrolytes, renal function tests, liver function tests, urinalysis, and blood cultures. Laboratory studies were normal with the exception of an elevated white blood cell count with lymphocytosis. During the first 24 hours of admission, her apneic events increased in frequency and consisted of cessation of breathing for 30 seconds or more, bradycardia, and cyanosis. She required transfer to the intensive care unit for mechanical ventilation. Ampicillin and gentamicin were initiated. Chest radiograph demonstrated "pulmonary vascular congestion."

Differential Diagnosis and Management

Apnea in a term infant may be the presenting symptom for systemic bacterial infection or sepsis, a cardiac arrhythmia, or seizure disorder. Other considerations include an anatomic abnormality (laryngomalacia or tracheomalacia) or failure of the central nervous system owing to head trauma or toxic overdose. Botulism should also be considered with accompanying epidemiology. Apnea also may be seen as a consequence of certain respiratory infections, most notably bronchiolitis caused by respiratory syncytial virus, influenza, and pertussis. Given the patient's rapid clinical deterioration, it is reasonable to suspect sepsis (even with the absence of fever) and initiate broad spectrum antibiotics to provide coverage for the most common etiologies (group B *Streptococcus*, *Escherichia* coli, and other gram-negative organisms). Additionally, it is reasonable to initiate a workup for other causes such as an electrocardiogram (EKG) to assess for a cardiac arrhythmia, and an electroencephalogram (EEG) to assess for seizure activity. Given the presence of nasal congestion and rhinorrhea, lymphcytosis, and pulmonary vascular congestion, a viral respiratory illness should also be strongly considered.

Case Presentation (continued)

The patient's condition did not significantly change over the subsequent 2 hospital days. Blood and urine cultures were negative, a respiratory viral PCR panel was negative, EKG revealed a normal sinus rhythm, and EEG did not show seizure activity. On hospital day 3 a *Bordetella pertussis* PCR was sent and returned as positive for *Bordetella pertussis*. Ampicillin and gentamicin were discontinued and the patient was started on a 5-day course of azithromycin. The resident physician caring for the patient calls hospital infection control for guidance on post-exposure prophylaxis.

Discussion and Control of Pertussis in Healthcare

Infection with *Bordetella pertussis*, the causative agent of pertussis (whooping cough), continues to be a significant cause of mortality and morbidity despite high vaccination coverage. According to the Centers of Disease Control and Prevention, there was a peak in the incidence of pertussis cases in 2004 (8.9 per 100,000) that was up from a low of 0.54 per 100,000 in 1981. The most recent data from 2008 shows that the incidence is 4.18 per 100,000, with a majority of the cases occurring in children less than 6 months of age, adolescents, and young adults. One of the reasons for this is because immunity conferred by vaccination wanes with increasing age, rendering many adolescents and adults susceptible to infection. Another reason is that pertussis often presents as a mild or atypical illness, which causes it to be overlooked in nonpediatric patients. Clinical symptoms result from the bacteria attaching to the cilia of the respiratory epithelial cells. Here, the bacteria produce a toxin that causes inflammation of the respiratory tract and paralysis of the cilia. This makes it difficult to clear secretions. Pertussis antigens appear to allow the organism to evade host defenses such that lymphocytosis is promoted but chemotaxis is impaired. The incubation period of pertussis is generally 7 to 10 days, with a range of 4 to 21 days. Rarely the incubation period may be as long as 42 days. The clinical course of illness is typically divided into three distinct stages; the catarrhal stage, lasting 1 to 2 weeks, which features coryza, sneezing, low grade fever, and mild cough; the paroxysmal stage, lasting 1 to 6 weeks, which features bursts or paroxysms of cough ending with a long inspiratory effort usually accompanied by a characteristic "whoop"; and the convalescent stage, lasting weeks to months which features a very gradual decrease of symptoms.

Secondary bacterial pneumonia, dehydration, anorexia, seizures, and encephalopathy are reported complications associated with pertussis, with pneumonia contributing the most towards pertussis-related deaths. Young infants are at highest risk for complications and death. Recent data among reported pertussis cases indicates that pneumonia occurred among nearly 12% of infants younger than 6 months, and among pertussis related deaths, 83% were in infants three months of age or younger.

Healthcare workers (HCWs) play a prominent role in the transmission of healthcare-associated pertussis. It is well known that, because of waning immunity, adult HCWs are a source of disease transmission. Wright et al. performed a retrospective cohort study measuring antibodies to pertussis toxin and fila-mentous hemagglutinin in the sera of resident physicians and emergency depart-ment employees at an academic medical center. They calculated the annual incidence in these populations to be 1.3% and 3.6%, respectively. Another study out of UCLA showed a higher incidence (33%) among its HCWs, although different antibody tests were used and the study was extended over a lon-ger period of time. Healthcare-associated pertussis can be transmitted among patients and HCWs creating the potential for a large number of infected indi-viduals. Neonates exposed to other infected patients or infected HCWs are at an increased risk of acquisition of illness, complications, and death. In 2010, a pertussis outbreak occurred in California where all but one of the ten pediatric deaths were among Hispanic infants less than 2 months of age.

The diagnosis of pertussis is based on clinical symptomatology as well as a positive laboratory test. Any symptomatic patient in whom pertussis is sus-pected should have a nasopharyngeal swab obtained and sent for *Bordetella pertussis* testing. A high index of suspicion should be held for neonates as they are at increased risk of mortality and morbidity. Culture has long been consid-ered the gold standard for laboratory diagnosis but its yield is often affected by poor specimen collection and transportation techniques. Additionally, because *B. pertussis* is fastidious, culture results may take several days to 2 weeks to become positive, obviating any clinical usefulness. PCR has increased sensitiv-ity and more rapid reporting and has become a widely employed test in many hospital labs. PCR testing may also be affected by poor specimen collection. Serologic testing may be useful in adolescents and adults who present later in the course of illness; however, a positive result may only represent previous exposure to *B. pertussis* and not necessarily acute infection.

There are a number of difficulties in controlling pertussis outbreaks and exposures in the healthcare environment despite the fact that we now have rapid PCR testing available. Again, pertussis is rarely considered in adults who present with prolonged cough, pertussis often presents as an atypical illness with mild symptoms, and adult HCWs take care of a highly susceptible patient population that is either unvaccinated (neonates) or has waning immunity (adult patients). To prevent transmission in the hospital setting, it is important to diagnose cases of pertussis promptly and to identify health care personnel and other patients that may have been exposed to known cases. Exposed per-sons should have symptoms monitored for 42 days after suspected exposure. If a patient is symptomatic, they should be placed under contact and droplet pre-cautions until they have completed five days of effective antimicrobial therapy or for 21 days after onset of cough if therapy is refused.

All patients and HCWs who are exposed to proven or probable cases of pertussis should be offered chemoprophylaxis to curtail disease transmission regardless of age or vaccination status.(Tables 8.3 and 8.4) Although erythro-mycin estolate remains the recommended agent, there are studies showing that azithromycin works just as well and is better tolerated. Azithromycin is recom-mended for neonates because of the risk of pyloric stenosis with erythromycin treatment. Exclusion of HCWs from work for the first 5 days of therapy is also recommended unless they refuse therapy, whereby they should be excluded for 21 days after cough onset. Asymptomatic persons need no exclusion.

Table 8.3 Treatment and Prevention of Pertussis (Whooping Cough)

Recommended treatment
• Macrolide antibiotic
• 5-day course of azithromycin
• 7-day course of clarithromycin
• 14-day course of erythromycin
• Alternate agent
• 14-day course of trimethoprim-sulfamethoxazole
• Treat persons aged >1 year within 3 weeks of cough onset
• Treat infants aged <1 year within 6 weeks of cough onset
Postexposure prophylaxis
• Administer course of antibiotic to close contacts within 3 weeks of exposure, especially in high-risk settings.
Prevention and surveillance
• Vaccinate children aged 6 weeks to 6 years with diphtheria, tetanus toxoids and acellular pertussis vaccine (DTaP). Give a single dose of Tetanus Toxoid and Reduced Diphtheria and Acellular Pertussis vaccine (Tdap) for adolescents and adults aged <65 years.
Report all cases to local and state health departments

Adapted from Tiwari, T, et al., Recommended antimicrobial agents for the treatment and postexposure prophylaxis of pertussis. 2005 CDC Guidelines. MMWR 2005;54(RR14):1–16.

Table 8.4 Close Contacts to Consider for Postexposure Prophylaxis

• A close contact of a patient with pertussis is a person who had face-to-face exposure within 3 feet of a symptomatic patient. Respiratory droplets (particles >5 µm in size) are generated during coughing, sneezing, or talking.
• Close contacts also can include persons who
• Have direct contact with respiratory, oral, or nasal secretions from a symptomatic patient
• Shared the same confined space in close proximity with a symptomatic patient for >1 hour
• Some close contacts are at high risk for acquiring severe disease following exposure to pertussis. These contacts include infants <1 year of age, persons with immunodeficiency syndromes, those with chronic lung disease, respiratory insufficiency, or cystic fibrosis.

Adapted from Tiwari T, et al. Recommended antimicrobial agents for the treatment and postexposure prophylaxis of pertussis. 2005 CDC Guidelines.MMWR 2005;54(RR14):1–16.

Vaccination offers a viable means of preventing pertussis in HCWs, especially those who work with children. Providing booster immunization to HCWs may help prevent transmission during hospital outbreaks. There have been studies of vaccination of HCWs during community or hospital outbreaks, but there are currently no official recommendations for use of vaccination in HCWs during outbreak situations.

Case Conclusion

The patient completed therapy of azithromycin and had slow respiratory improvement. She was extubated on hospital day 9 and was discharged from the hospital after 12 days. Twenty-four HCWs and three patients were identified as having significant exposure to the pertussis patient during the period when illness was not suspected and she remained unisolated. All patients had up to date vaccination status and 18 of the HCWs had received a Tdap booster in adulthood given their occupation of working among neonates, infants, and children. Twenty HCWs and all three exposed patients accepted postexposure prophylaxis and four HCWs did not. One HCW who refused prophylaxis and who had not received a Tdap booster developed a respiratory illness that was confirmed by PCR to be due to *B. pertussis* and was furloughed for 21 days. No other illness was identified among the contacts.

Suggested Reading

Centers for Disease Control and Prevention. Epidemiology and Prevention of Vaccine-Preventable Diseases. Atkinson W, Wolfe S, Hamborsky J, eds. 12th ed. Washington, DC: Public Health Foundation, 2011.

CDC. Guidelines for the control of pertussis outbreaks. Atlanta, GA: Centers for Disease Control and Prevention, 2000.

Christie CD et al. A trial of acellular pertussis vaccine in hospital workers during the Cincinnati pertussis epidemic of 1993. Clin Infect Dis 2001;33(7):997–1003.

Deville JG et al. Frequency of unrecognized Bordetella pertussis infections in adults. Clin Infect Dis 1995;21(3):639–642.

Guiso N et al. The Global Pertussis Initiative: report from a round table meeting to discuss the epidemiology and detection of pertussis, Paris, France, 11–12 January 2010. Vaccine 2011;29(6):1115–1121.

Hall-Baker PA et al. Summary of notifiable diseases - United States, 2008. MMWR Morb Mortal Weekly Rep 2010;57(54):1–94.

Langley JM et al. Azithromycin is as effective as and better tolerated than erythromycin estolate for the treatment of pertussis. Pediatrics 2004;114(1):e96–101.

Lavine J et al. Imperfect vaccine-induced immunity and whooping cough transmission to infants. Vaccine 2010;29(1):11–16.

Outbreaks of pertussis associated with hospitals--Kentucky, Pennsylvania, and Oregon, 2003. MMWR Morb Mortal Wkly Rep 2005;54(3):67–71.

Shefer A et al. Use and safety of acellular pertussis vaccine among adult hospital staff during an outbreak of pertussis. J Infect Dis 1995;171(4):1053–1056.

Tiwari T et al. Recommended antimicrobial agents for the treatment and postexposure prophylaxis of pertussis. 2005 CDC Guidelines. MMWR Morbid Mortal Wkly Rep 2005;54(RR-14):1–16.

Winter K, Harriman K, Schechter R, Yamada E, Talarico DO, Chavez G, California Dept of Public Health. Pertussis—California, January–June 2010. MMWR Morb Mortal Wkly Rep 2010;59(26):817.

Wright SW, Decker MD, Edwards KM. Incidence of pertussis infection in healthcare workers. Infect Control Hosp Epidemiol 1999;20(2):120–123.

Chapter 8c

Respiratory Syncytial Virus in the Neonatal Intensive Care Unit

Sandra Fowler

Case Presentation

Baby Boy KC was delivered in early December by caesarean section at 27 weeks gestation due to maternal preterm labor and twin gestation. Birth weight was 1120 grams. He received intratracheal surfactant, but required mechanical ventilation on the first day of life for respiratory failure, and was treated for presumed sepsis with a 7-day course of ampicillin and gentamicin. He was weaned rapidly to nasal continuous positive airway pressure (CPAP) on day of life two, and then to nasal cannula oxygen by day of life 29. He was weaned to room air on day of life 46, and was growing and gaining weight on full enteral feeds. On the evening of day of life 47, he developed episodes of apnea and bradycardia with accompanying desaturations and was placed on nasal CPAP. His exam showed upper airway congestion, mild subcostal retractions, but no wheezing. A sepsis workup was performed and the infant was started on nafcillin and gentamicin. The endotracheal aspirate showed moderate WBC, few epithelial cells, and no organisms. Chest radiograph was unremarkable. Rapid respiratory syncytial virus (RSV) testing was negative. A respiratory viral PCR panel was sent. By day of life 51, he developed increasing tachypnea, retractions, and CO_2 retention, and appeared pale and mottled. He was intubated and mechanically ventilated, and had placement of an arterial line. His respiratory acidosis worsened, requiring high frequency jet ventilation, and he was retreated again with surfactant. The respiratory viral PCR panel returned positive for RSV on day of life 53.

Differential Diagnosis and Management

Nosocomial bacterial or fungal sepsis with or without pneumonia is certainly a consideration in this patient, though less likely because of fact that the infant had not been intubated in 20 days, had no recent broad spectrum antibiotics, was on full feeds, and had no central line. His cultures remained negative, and the endotracheal aspirate did not suggest a bacterial pneumonia. Respiratory viruses, including influenza, RSV, adenovirus, and parainfluenza, are compatible with the initial presentation of apnea and increased upper airway congestion, as is the onset of illness during the winter months.

RSV is a ubiquitous pathogen of childhood, infecting nearly all children by two years of age. Infection is seasonal in temperate climates, occurring in winter and early spring, but occurs year round in the tropics. In the otherwise healthy infant and child, illness is characterized by nasal congestion, cough, wheezing, increased work of breathing, poor feeding, fever, and may be associated with low oxygen saturation. Infection in the preterm infant, however, may produce few signs of respiratory tract disease. These infants may initially present with lethargy, irritability, feeding intolerance, and apnea. Potential risk factors for nosocomial infection due to RSV include prematurity, lung disease, heart disease and immunosuppression. Infants with underlying lung or congenital heart disease are at particular risk for respiratory failure or pulmonary hypertension as complications of infection.

Transmission occurs via exposure to large droplets at short distance, and by fomites. In the hospital setting, transmission most likely occurs by inoculation into the eye or nose from contaminated hands of care givers or visitors or from fomites. The incubation period ranges between two to eight days. Shedding of virus may occur for up to four weeks in infected neonates. The transmission of RSV within the hospital by healthcare providers is common. One report estimated that more than 40% of staff working on a children's ward acquired RSV during a 2-month period of increased community RSV activity (and thus subsequent increased hospital admissions for RSV) and 27% of patients under their care were thought to have acquired infection while in the hospital Additionally, more than 50% of staff acquired RSV on average 18 to 19 days after admission of the first patient with RSV to their ward. This underscores the importance of healthcare workers taking appropriate precautions when they have respiratory symptoms. Suggestions have ranged from use of masks, gloves, and gowns for patient care to furlough of staff until respiratory symptoms have resolved. Individual wards or units may develop staff policies which take into account the patient population at risk.

Diagnosis of RSV is confirmed by enzyme immunoassay or direct immunofluorescence of nasal secretions, or by PCR testing of nasal secretions. The sensitivity of antigen detection assays is generally between 80% and 90%, whereas that of PCR approaches 100% for nasopharyngeal aspirates. Multiplex respiratory virus PCR testing is now available at many hospitals and is able to identify other viral respiratory pathogens in addition to RSV.

Case Presentation (continued)

The infant continued to have severe respiratory acidosis until day of life 58, when he was weaned to conventional ventilation. He was extubated and weaned to nasal cannula oxygen on day of life 60. He was otherwise doing well at that time except for slow growth velocity. He was ultimately weaned to room air, except during feedings, and was discharged home in February on day of life 73. He returned to the outpatient clinic in March for an injection of palivizumab.

Treatment of RSV is generally supportive and may include provision of supplemental oxygen, nasal suctioning, and management of respiratory failure using mechanical ventilation as necessary. Aerosolized ribavirin has shown activity against RSV, but has not been shown to reduce the need for mechanical ventilation. Lack of significant clinical benefit, along with the potential toxicity and difficulty in administration limit its usefulness in the NICU setting. Inhaled beta-adrenergic agents may be effective in some infants, but should not be continued in infants who do not show an initial response. Corticosteroids have not been shown to be beneficial. Prophylaxis of at risk infants using a humanized monoclonal antibody, palivizumab, is effective in preventing severe disease, and is routinely prescribed at discharge for premature infants with certain risk profiles, and for infants with certain types of chronic lung disease and congenital heart defects as a once monthly injection given throughout the RSV season. Infants who are eligible for prophylaxis continue to be at risk throughout RSV season even after experiencing infection. Palivizumab has no role in the treatment of established RSV disease.

Nosocomial transmission of RSV is less common in the NICU than on general pediatric wards, but poses additional challenges in prevention, control, and costs, both in health outcomes among vulnerable infants, and in dollars expended to contain spread of infection. Costs to care for infected infants and to contain spread in one NICU outbreak amounted to over 1 million dollars in direct hospital charges, plus costs associated with disruption of unit activity, surveillance, and prophylaxis.

In addition to practicing standard precautions, infants with RSV should be placed in contact and droplet precautions. Caregivers should practice hand hygiene after contact with the patient or fomites. Gowns and gloves should be worn when entering the patient's environment of care, which may consist of a separate room in the NICU, or a designated area within an open unit. A surgical mask and eye protection, or a face shield should be worn when performing any procedure likely to generate sprays of respiratory secretions. Other measures that may be used in the outbreak setting include screening of other infants in the NICU, and cohorting those who are infected, along with the staff caring for them (Table 8.5). The Centers for Disease Control has not made a recommendation for the use of anti-RSV monoclonal antibody (palivizumab) to control outbreaks of RSV; however, there is limited data describing the successful use of palivizumab in limiting NICU outbreaks of RSV.

Case Conclusion

Another infant, who was located in a crib next to the case infant developed congestion and cough and was immediately placed in contact and droplet precautions. The rapid RSV was returned positive on this infant 2 days later. These two infants remained in contact and droplet precautions for 21 days. Other infants in the same area were observed for any signs of respiratory viral infection and placed in contact and droplet precautions for 7 days. No other infants

Table 8.5 Infection Control Measures Evaluated for Prevention of Viral Nosocomial Infection Including RSV in Neonatal Intensive Care Units

General Measures Most Commonly Adopted

Rapid screening diagnostic tests upon admission to hospital or specialty care unit

Hand hygiene with alcohol-based hand rubs or soap and water

Cohorting of infected patients

Glove use when entering patient room and changing between patients; decontaminate hands after glove removal

Gown use when entering patient room and change after each patient contact avoiding contact of contaminated gown with clothes

Mask and eye protection use when performing procedures or patient-care activities that might generate sprays of respiratory secretions

Cohorting of healthcare staff

Limit visits by family members and ensure that visitors obey appropriate infection containment procedures.

Specific for RSV

Consider prophylactic palivizumab to contacts of infected patients when other containment measures fail.

RSV, respiratory syncytial virus.

Adapted by permission from Macmillan Publishers Ltd: Groothuis J, Bauman J, Malinoski F, Eggleston M. Strategies for prevention of RSV nosocomial infection. J Perinatol 2008;28:319–323, copyright 2008.

were moved into the area during this time. Staff were educated regarding transmission of RSV, but were not cohorted with the affected infants. Unit visitation was not restricted. There were no additional RSV cases in the NICU.

Suggested Reading

Groothuis J, Bauman J, Malinoski F, Eggleston M. Strategies for prevention of RSV nosocomial infection. J Perinatol 2008;28:319–323.

Halasa N, Williams J, Wilson G, Walsh W, Schaffner W, Wright P. Medical and economic impact of a respiratory syncytial virus outbreak in a neonatal intensive care unit. Pediatr Infect Dis J. 2005;24:1040–1044.

Kurz H, Herbach K, Janata O, Sterniste W, Bauer K. Experience with the use of palivizumab together with infection control measures to prevent respiratory syncytial virus outbreaks in neonatal intensive care units. J Hosp Infect 2008;70:246–252.

Respiratory Syncytial Virus. In: Pickering LK, ed. Red Book. Elk Grove Village, IL: American Academy of Pediatrics, 2009.

Tablon O, Anderson L, Besser R, Bridges C, Hajjeh R. Guidelines for preventing healthcare-associated pneumonia, 2003. MMWR Morbid Mortal Wkly Rep. 2004;53(RR-03):1–36.

Chapter 9a

The Methicillin-Resistant Staphylococcus aureus-Colonized Patient

Jeremy Storm and Daniel Diekema

Case Presentation

A 76 year old female long-term care facility (LTCF) resident with a history of diabetes mellitus, hypertension, depression, and mild dementia is brought to the hospital after being found on the floor of her room unable to walk, with right leg pain and mental status changes. In the emergency department, she was afebrile but was hypotensive (blood pressure of 88/40), tachycardic to 110, and had a respiratory rate of 24 per minute. She was confused and her right leg was shortened and externally rotated. Her hemoglobin was 7.2, head computerized tomography and electrocardiogram were normal, and radiographs of the right hip confirmed a right femoral neck fracture. The patient was given a fluid bolus and 2 units of packed red blood cells, transferred to the intensive care unit (ICU), and orthopedic surgery was consulted. As per hospital protocol for patients transferred from other healthcare facilities, including LTCFs, a rapid nares screen for methicillin-resistant *Staphylococcus aureus* (MRSA) was obtained in the emergency department and was positive (Fig. 9.1).

Because of her hemodynamic instability, she was admitted to the ICU and because of her MRSA colonization status, she was placed in a private room and on contact precautions (standard precautions plus a gown and gloves for all contact with the patient or patient's immediate environment). She was evaluated by orthopedic surgery, who recommended hip arthroplasty as soon as the patient was clinically stable. Infectious Diseases was consulted at the request of orthopedics, to make recommendations regarding possible MRSA decolonization prior to surgery and to optimize choice of perioperative antibiotics.

Initial Management

Staphylococcus aureus can be a devastating healthcare-associated pathogen, and is the most common cause of surgical site infections. Approximately half of all healthcare-associated *S. aureus* infections are caused by MRSA, making MRSA the most common multiple-drug resistant organism (MDRO) in U.S. hospitals. Most *S. aureus* infections are endogenous, caused by the same strain colonizing

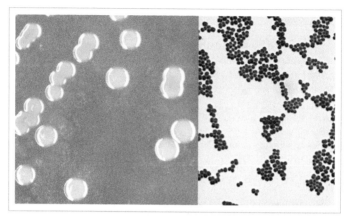

Figure 9.1 *Left*: Colonies of methicillin-resistant *Staphylococcus aureus* (MRSA) on a chromogenic agar plate used for nares screening. *Right*: Gram stain of MRSA colony.

an individual (usually in the nares, but also other body sites such as the throat and GI tract). Moreover, *S. aureus* (including MRSA) carriers are known to be at a greater risk than noncarriers for *S. aureus* infection during receipt of health care. As a result, prevention of MRSA infections is currently focused on: (1) preventing those who are not colonized from acquiring the organism, and (2) preventing those who are colonized with MRSA from becoming infected.

For prevention of MDRO transmission, the CDC recommends the addition of contact precautions (CP) to standard precautions for those known to be infected with, or colonized by, an MDRO (including MRSA). The evidence supporting CP for prevention of MDRO transmission is largely based on the success of this approach from uncontrolled observational studies, many of which have been conducted in the setting of an outbreak or during periods of "hyperendemic" (elevated) rates of an MDRO combined with microbiological studies demonstrating MDRO contamination of the patient environment—including the clothing of individuals who have close contact with that environment. Because the minority of MRSA-colonized patients are detected by clinical cultures, some recommend "active detection" by sampling the nares of uninfected patients, in order to identify those who are colonized so that CP can be initiated and/or to implement a decolonization program. This active detection and isolation (ADI) approach has been intensely debated, given that studies performed among different patient populations and utilizing different ADI strategies have reported conflicting results. Additionally, there is the potential for unintended adverse consequences of broad application of CP (e.g., less contact with healthcare providers, higher rates of anxiety and depression, lower satisfaction with care, etc.). Identifying the MRSA-colonized patient can also be a challenge, because MRSA may reside in the nares, skin (especially wounds), oropharynx and gastrointestinal tract. Therefore, performing only a nares culture or PCR test may miss a substantial proportion of colonization (up to 30% in some studies).

The CDC/HICPAC guideline suggests ADI as a Tier 2 intervention, to be considered during MRSA outbreaks or when the rate of MRSA infection is stable or rising despite assiduous application of standard infection prevention (Tier 1) approaches (Table 9.1) Nonetheless, some states and healthcare systems (e.g., Veteran's Affairs) have mandated the use of ADI for acute care facilities. As a result, MRSA screening practices vary substantially from one facility to another in the United States, as do approaches to CP and decolonization. Many hospitals, such as the one to which this patient was admitted, apply ADI only to patients considered to be at highest risk of MRSA colonization (e.g., LTCF residents, transfers from other healthcare facilities, and patients with a history of MRSA colonization or infection).

For prevention of MRSA infection among those already colonized, the focus should be on the application of bundled practices to prevent device associated infections (e.g., CLABSI, VAP), and on the use of surface decolonization to lower the colonizing organism burden. For SSI prevention, a recent randomized controlled trial suggested that the use of chlorhexidine (CHG) bathing and intranasal mupirocin among known *S. aureus* carriers substantially reduced the *S. aureus* SSI rate. Although the study included no MRSA carriers, there is biological plausibility to apply this finding to this population.

The most commonly used MRSA decolonization regimen is mupirocin 2% nasal ointment (applied twice daily for at least 5 days) combined with daily CHG bathing. This regimen is successful at eradicating MRSA nasal carriage temporarily in over 80% of patients, but many of these will recolonize over time. Therefore, decolonization is best applied immediately prior to a defined risk period (e.g., perioperatively to prevent SSI) or to interrupt transmission during outbreaks, and is not recommended as a routine "Tier 1" measure by CDC (see Table 9.1). One reason to limit the use of decolonization is the potential for emergence of resistance to the agents used.

Case Presentation (continued)

The patient responded well to supportive care and pain control, with stabilization of vital signs and improvement in mental status. The infectious disease consultant recommended application of mupirocin twice daily to the nares, and daily chlorhexidine body washes, to begin immediately and continue perioperatively. For perioperative antibiotic prophylaxis, a single dose of vancomycin was recommended and administered approximately 60 minutes prior to the first incision.

The hip replacement was uneventful, and by postoperative day five the patient was able to ambulate short distances with assistance and was therefore discharged to the rehabilitation unit affiliated with her LTCF. A follow up MRSA nares screen prior to discharge was negative. She was seen in follow-up by orthopedic surgery at 4 weeks after discharge, and was found to be doing well, with no evidence of infection and good prosthesis function.

However, when the patient was admitted 6 months later for chest pain evaluation, she again tested positive for MRSA nares colonization and was placed into CP. During this hospitalization, she became increasingly anxious

Table 9.1 Summary of Tier 1 and Tier 2 Recommendations for Prevention and Control of MDROs in Healthcare Settings

Category	Tier 1: For ROUTINE implementation	Tier 2: For INTENSIFIED control efforts
Administrative Support and Adherence Monitoring	• Make MDRO prevention and control an organizational priority • Provide administrative support ($$ and personnel) • Identify experts who can provide consultation • Implement communication systems • Implement process to monitor and improve HCP adherence to recommended practices • Implement systems to designate patients known to be colonized/infected with an MDRO • Support participation in local, regional and/or national coalitions to combat MDROs • Provide updated feedback at least annually to healthcare providers and administrators	• Obtain expert consultation from persons with experience in infection control and MDROs • Provide necessary leadership, funding, and day-to-day oversight to implement interventions selected • Evaluate healthcare system factors for role in creating or perpetuating MDRO transmission (e.g., staffing levels, communication processes) • Update healthcare providers and administrators on the progress and effectiveness of the intensified interventions
MDRO Education	• Provide education and training on MDRO transmission prevention during orientation for healthcare personnel (HCP), with periodic updates	• Intensify the frequency of educational programs, especially for those who work in areas where MDRO rates are not decreasing
Judicious Antimicrobial Use	• Ensure that a multi-disciplinary process is in place to foster appropriate antimicrobial use • Implement systems to prompt clinicians to use the appropriate agent for the given situation • Provide clinicians with susceptibility reports and analysis of trends, updated at least annually	• Review the role of antimicrobial use in perpetuating the MDRO problem targeted for intensified intervention • Control and improve antimicrobial use as indicated

Surveillance	• Use standardized laboratory methods and published guidelines for determining antimicrobial susceptibilities of MDROs	• Calculate and analyze incidence rates of target MDROs
	• Establish systems to ensure that clinical labs promptly notify infection prevention when a novel resistance pattern is detected	• Increase frequency of compiling, monitoring antimicrobial susceptibility summary reports
	• Develop and implement lab protocols for storing isolates of MDROs for molecular typing	• Perform typing of target MDRO if needed
	• Establish laboratory-based systems to detect and communicate evidence of MDROs in clinical isolates	• Develop and implement protocols to obtain active surveillance cultures from patients in populations at risk.
	• Prepare facility-specific antimicrobial susceptibility reports as recommended by CLSI	• Conduct culture surveys to assess efficacy of intensified MDRO control interventions.
	• Monitor reports for evidence of changing resistance that may indicate emergence or transmission of MDROs	• Conduct serial unit specific point prevalence culture surveys of the target MDRO to determine if transmission has decreased or ceased
	• Develop and monitor special-care unit-specific antimicrobial susceptibility reports	• Repeat point-prevalence culture surveys at routine intervals until transmission has ceased
	• Monitor trends in incidence of target MDROs in the facility over time	• If indicated by assessment of the MDRO problem, collect cultures to assess the colonization status of patients with substantial exposure to those with known MDRO infection or colonization
		• Obtain cultures from HCP for target MDROs when there is epidemiologic evidence implicating the staff member as a source of ongoing transmission

(continued)

Table 9.1 (Continued)

Category	Tier 1: For ROUTINE implementation	Tier 2: For INTENSIFIED control efforts
Infection Control Precautions to Prevent Transmission	• Follow Standard Precautions in all healthcare settings • In acute care setting, follow Contact Precautions for all patients known to be colonized/infected with MDROs (for other healthcare settings). • When single-patient rooms are available, assign priority for these rooms to patients with known or suspected MDRO colonization or infection • When single-patient rooms are not available, cohort patients with the same MDRO in the same room or patient-care area • When cohorting patients with the same MDRO is not possible, place MDRO patients in rooms with patients who are at low risk for MDRO acquisition and associated adverse outcomes from infection.	• Implement Contact Precautions (CP) routinely for all patients colonized or infected with a target MDRO • Don gowns and gloves before or upon entry to the patient's room or cubicle • When active surveillance cultures are obtained as part of an intensified MDRO control program, implement CP until the surveillance culture is reported negative for the target MDRO • No recommendation is made for universal use of gloves and/or gowns. (Unresolved issue) • Implement policies for patient admission and placement as needed to prevent transmission of the problem MDRO • Stop new admissions to the unit/facility if transmission continues despite intensified control measures
Environmental Measures	• Follow recommended cleaning, disinfection and sterilization guidelines for maintaining patient care areas and equipment • Dedicate noncritical medical items to use on individual patients known to be infected or colonized with an MDRO • Prioritize room cleaning of patients on Contact Precautions • Focus on cleaning and disinfecting frequently touched surfaces and equipment in immediate vicinity of patient.	• Implement patient dedicated use of non-critical equipment • Intensify and reinforce training of environmental staff who work in areas targeted for intensified MDRO control • Monitor cleaning performance to ensure consistent cleaning and disinfection of surfaces in close proximity to the patient and those likely to be touched by the patient and HCWs • Obtain environmental cultures (e.g., surfaces, shared equipment) only when epidemiologically implicated in transmission • Vacate units for environmental assessment and intensive cleaning when previous efforts to control environmental transmission have failed

Decolonization	• Not recommended routinely	• Consult with experts on a case-by-case basis regarding the appropriate use of decolonization therapy for patients or staff during a limited period of time as a component of an intensified MRSA control program
		• When decolonization for MRSA is used, perform susceptibility testing for the decolonizing agent against the target organism or the MDRO strain epidemiologically implicated in transmission.
		• Monitor susceptibility to detect emergence of resistance to the decolonizing agent
		• Limit decolonization to HCP found to be colonized with MRSA who have been epidemiologically implicated in ongoing transmission of MRSA to patients

HCP, healthcare personnel.

Adapted from Table 3 in Siegel JD, Rhinehart E, Jackson M, Chiarello L and the Healthcare Infection Control Practices Advisory Committee. 2006. Management of multidrug-resistant organisms in healthcare settings. 2006. Am J Infect Control 2007;35(10 Suppl 2):S165–193. Available at: http://www.cdc.gov/ncidod/dhqp/pdf/ar/mdroGuideline2006.pdf.

and paranoid, and required transfer to the medicine-psychiatry unit for management of depression symptoms in the setting of dementia. Her clinicians judged that her CP status was too "isolating," and was therefore impeding her care. In consultation with the infectious diseases service and the infection prevention program, she was removed from CP for the remainder of her hospitalization, provided she developed no signs or symptoms of active infection.

Management

This case highlights the complexity of several issues related to the MRSA colonized patient, including MRSA ADI, MRSA decolonization, perioperative antibiotic selection for MRSA colonized patients, and posthospitalization follow up of those identified as being colonized with MRSA. Every hospital must aggressively seek to prevent MDRO transmission, and the measures used will vary according to the epidemiology of each MDRO at a given hospital. In addition, allowances may need to be made for individual patients in whom special circumstances apply—for example, during this patient's readmission the risks of CP were felt to outweigh the potential benefits. If she had been actively infected with a draining wound, the risk-benefit calculation may have been different. Similarly, the use of CP for all colonized patients in LTCFs is not appropriate, given that LTCFs serve as a patient's residence, and consideration must be given for social interaction and group activities.

This case also illustrates the increasingly common practice of S. aureus decolonization as an approach to SSI prevention, and demonstrates that many decolonized patients will re-colonize over time. If this SSI prevention approach becomes standard of care, monitoring for the emergence of resistance to the topical antimicrobial agents employed (e.g., CHG and mupirocin) will become increasingly important. The additional advantage of knowing the S. aureus/MRSA colonization status of a surgical patient is also illustrated here: it allows for adjustment of perioperative antimicrobial prophylaxis to include anti-MRSA coverage if necessary. An alternative approach that wouldn't require screening would be to base perioperative antimicrobial decisions on the local epidemiology of SSI (proportion due to methicillin resistant organisms, risk factors among surgical patients, etc.).

Case Conclusion

The rest of this patient's second admission was uneventful, and she was discharged back to her LTCF in good condition. At her LTCF, the infection control policy recommended CP for MRSA colonized patients only if they had an active infection or draining wound. Thus, she was not placed in CP, and was allowed to socialize and participate in group activities at her LTCF, which she greatly enjoyed.

Suggested Reading

Bode LG, Kluytmans JA, Wertheim HF, et al. Preventing surgical site infections in nasal carriers of Staphylococcus aureus. NEJM 2010;362:9–17.

Cooper BS, Stone SP, Kibbler CC, Cookson BD, Roberts JA, Medley GF, et al. Systematic review of isolation policies in the hospital management of methicillin-resistant *Staphylococcus aureus*: a review of the literature with epidemiological and economic modeling. Health Technol Assess 2003;7:1–194.

Morgan DJ, Diekema DJ, Sepkowitz K, Perencevich EN. Adverse outcomes associated with contact precautions: A review of the literature. Am J Infect Control 2009;37:85–93.

Peterson LR, Diekema DJ. To screen or not to screen for MRSA. J Clin Microbiol 2010;48:683–89.

Siegel JD, Rhinehart E, Jackson M, Chiarello L, and the Healthcare Infection Control Practices Advisory Committee. 2006. Management of multidrug-resistant organisms in healthcare settings, 2006. Am J Infect Control 2007;35(10 Suppl 2):S165–193. Available at: http://www.cdc.gov/ncidod/dhqp/pdf/ar/mdroGuideline2006.pdf.

Weber SG, Huang SS, Oriola S, Huskins WC, Noskin GA, Harriman K, et al. Legislative mandates for use of active surveillance cultures to screen for methicillin-resistant *Staphylococcus aureus* and vancomycin-resistant enterococci: position statement from the joint SHEA and APIC Task Force. Infect Control Hosp Epidemiol 2007;28:249–60.

Chapter 9b

Highly Resistant Gram-Negative Bacteria

Dror Marchaim and Keith Kaye

Initial Case Presentation

An 84-year-old woman was admitted to the medicine floor 4 days ago with mild exacerbation of congestive heart failure, pulmonary edema, and a mildly elevated serum troponin. The patient usually resides in an advanced-care nursing home facility and suffers from progressive dementia. The patient is incontinent of stool and urine, and requires assistance in all activities of daily living. Additional comorbid conditions include diabetes, hypertension, decubitus pressure ulcers (grade III-IV), and a recent cerebral vascular event resulting in left-sided hemiplegia. At the time of admission, the treating physician ordered that a urinary catheter be inserted in order to monitor urine output. The urinary catheter was removed yesterday (hospital day 3). On morning rounds today, the patient seems weaker than usual, and the nurse reports that she hasn't eaten well in the past day. The patient is responsive, but is less alert than her baseline state. She is afebrile, blood pressure is 138/92 mmHg, heart rate is 89 beats/min, and there are no significant new findings on physical examination. A urinary catheter is reinserted, and a urine dipstick examination of a sample obtained from the catheter reveals pyuria, with microscopic evidence of numerous bacteria that appear to be gram-negative bacilli after staining. Urine culture and blood cultures are obtained, and the patient is started on antimicrobial therapy with intravenous cefepime and vancomycin.

After 48 hours on antibiotics (hospital day 6), the patient remains an inpatient on the medical floor, with an indwelling urinary catheter. She remains afebrile. The urine culture demonstrates growth of more than 10^5 colony forming units of *Klebsiella pneumoniae*, which is resistant to all β-lactam antibiotics (except piperacillin-tazobactam [MIC = 4 μg/ml]), cephalosporins (including ceftriaxone, ceftazidime, and cefepime), fluoroquinolones, and amikacin. The isolate is susceptible to tobramycin, colistin, tigecycline, ertapenem (MIC = 2 μg/ml), and meropenem (MIC = 1 μg/ml). The extended-spectrum β-lactamase (ESBL) phenotypic test is positive according to the automated microbiology laboratory system. Blood cultures continue to demonstrate no growth.

Differential Diagnosis and Initial Management

Based on the absence of new signs or symptoms of infection as well as the results of urine culture, the patient appears to have asymptomatic bacteriuria. Based on the available evidence, antimicrobial treatment for asymptomatic bacteriuria offers little to no benefit for virtually any hospitalized patient. This remains the case irrespective of which specific pathogen is isolated. Therefore, in this case, antibiotics should be discontinued promptly. Nonetheless, the finding of a highly resistant pathogen as a colonizing strain still has important management implications and serves as the basis for the remainder of this discussion.

Although treatment with antibiotics is not necessary, this patient has been identified as a carrier of a gram negative isolate that produces a β-lactamase resistance enzyme. Determining the pattern of resistance (if not the specific mechanism) is important not only in facilitating the selection of appropriate antimicrobial coverage when appropriate, but should also influence decisions about the most appropriate infection control precautions. Extended spectrum ESBL-producing strains are typically resistant to a range of β-lactam and cephalosporin agents. In addition, such strains may not reliably respond to treatment with β-lactam/β-lactamase inhibitors such as piperacillin-tazobactam (even though susceptibility to such combinations can be used to identify such isolates in the lab).

In this case, the organism should be specifically tested for carbapenemase production using the Hodge test (Fig. 9.2) or PCR-based techniques. Initial laboratory reports cannot otherwise reliably differentiate between carbapenemases and extended spectrum beta lactamase (ESBL) enzymes. If an *Enterobacteriaceae* has an MIC of 1 μg/ml or greater to meropenem, imipenem or doripenem; or an MIC of 2 μg/ml or greater to ertapenem, then a clinician should be suspicious that the organism is a carbapenem-resistant enterobacteriaceae (CRE).

Some hospitals have adopted policies that specifically recommend contact isolation precautions for patients who are infected or colonized with ESBL-producing organisms, although routine use of such precautions for ESBL-producing pathogens remains controversial. Contact isolation (the donning of gowns and gloves for contact with the patient and immediate environment) has been demonstrated to reduce patient-to-patient transmission of pathogens in the hospital (particularly in outbreak settings). However, the impact of contact precautions in preventing spread of endemic (established) disease is less certain.

One approach to balance these competing considerations is to employ contact precautions only for patients colonized or infected with pathogens deemed to be a more significant threat to patients at a given hospital (based on epidemiological and clinical trends). These priorities might vary from institution to institution. For example, CRE represent an especially serious threat to infection control and clinical management in most centers because there are limited therapeutic options available for infections caused by these exceptionally resistant pathogens. In many cases, CREs are susceptible only to polymixins (which are nephrotoxic), aminoglycosides (which are also nephrotoxic and are usually not recommended for monotherapy of serious infections) and tigecycline (which due to pharmacodynamic properties is suboptimal for treating bacteremia). In

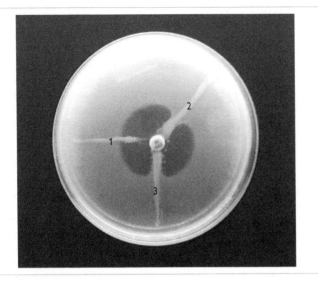

Figure 9.2 Results of the Modified Hodge Test for 3 Test Strains of
Enterobacteriaceae
A carbapenem disk is placed on the plate with susceptible *E.coli*. Three test strains
of *Enterobacteriaceae* (1–3) are individually streaked onto the plate. A positive result
reveals a cloverleaf-like indentation in the area of the susceptible *E. coli* which is growing
within the disk diffusion zone and indicates that the tested organism produces a carbapenemase. In this image, strains 2 and 3 appear to produce a carbapenemase.

(Photograph courtesy of Hussein Salimnia, PhD, Detroit Medical Center, MI, USA.)

some instances, CRE are resistant to all antimicrobials tested. Thus, in most all
circumstances, patients colonized with CRE should be subjected to strict contact precautions. For extra caution, in some instances, such patients have been
cohorted on a special hospital unit with dedicated staff in order to absolutely
minimize the risk for transmission of these pathogens. Rates of CRE should be
closely monitored in hospitals and microbiology laboratories. Additional strategies and recommendations for controlling CRE spread in hospitals are detailed
in recent recommendations from the U.S. Centers for Disease Control and
Prevention (Table 9.2).

Misuse and overuse of antimicrobial agents represent an important risk for
the emergence of highly resistant gram-negative pathogens. Therefore, another
important consideration in limiting the spread of such resistance in the hospital
is to limit the use of specific carbapenems, including imipenem, meropenem
and doripenem. When carbapenem therapy is absolutely necessary, such as for
treatment of invasive infections due to ESBL-producing organisms, a carbapenem lacking antipseudomonal activity such as ertapenem should be considered. Ertapenem theoretically will impart less selective antimicrobial pressure
than other drugs from the class with a broader spectrum of activity. However,
well-controlled clinical data to support this presumption are lacking.

Table 9.2 Principles and Recommendations for Optimal Control and Prevention of Spread of Carbapenem-Resistant or Carbapenemase-Producing *Enterobacteriaceae* in Hospitals

Parameter	Remarks
Contact precautions	Gown and gloves, single patient room if possible, appropriate signage
Enhanced adherence to hand hygiene proper practices	Conducting observations and interventions to improve adherence
Cohorting of patients	Dedicated staff contributes further to impact of cohorting
Microbiology testing for carbapenemase production [a]	Screening ESBL-producing *Enterobacteriaceae* and isolates with elevated MIC to ertapenem (≥2 mg/ml) for carbapenemase production using modified Hodge test or PCR-based methodology
Notification of every CRE case to Infection Control stuff	Clinical microbiology laboratory should establish strict protocol for testing and reporting
Point prevalence cultures in high-risk units	Particularly useful during epidemics or sudden increases in endemic rates
Active surveillance cultures policy of high risk patients	Examples: (1) new admissions from certain long-term care institutions if the rates in these institutions are known to be high, (2) patients from a high risk hospital location (e.g. burn unit) who stayed in close proximity to a CRE case.
Review microbiology records for the preceding year to determine whether CRE cases might have been missed	Particularly useful when CRE are not yet endemic in the region / facility
Monitor rates of CRE in the facility	Should be a priority of Infection Control and Prevention personnel
Implement antimicrobial stewardship programs in the facility	Focus on limiting the use of carbapenems, other broad-spectrum agents, and misuse of antibiotics in general
Establish communication with referral facilities	Specifically high risk facilities like LTACs; transfer of patients with CRE should be communicated prior to transfer
Enhance Infection Control practices in nearby non-tertiary-academic facilities	Infection Control practitioners should "reach-out" to neighboring institutions to help improve infection control practices across the healthcare continuum
Enforcement and monitoring of cleaning practices	Effective terminal cleaning of patients; rooms, conduct observations to assure that adequate cleaning practices are being utilized

ESBL, extended-spectrum β-lactamase; LTAC, long-term acute care facility; MIC, minimal inhibitory concentration.
[a] New CLSI criteria (Clinical and Laboratory Standard Institutes) state that carbapenemase producing testing are not mandatory if lower breakpoints are applied.

After the treating physician is informed of the results of the urine culture, he asks that an Infectious Diseases (ID) specialist see the patient. The consultant recommends discontinuation of the systemic antibiotics and immediate removal of the urinary catheter. While awaiting results of the Hodge test, the patient is moved to a private room and contact precautions are implemented. The next day, the laboratory reports the Hodge test to be positive, indicating that the organism is a CRE. The patient is clinically stable and is discharged back to her long-term care facility (LTCF). The LTCF is contacted and informed that the patient was identified as colonized with CRE. In addition, the patient is "flagged" in the hospital's computerized system, so that at the time of future admissions, she will be identified as a CRE carrier and subjected to strict isolation precautions pending subsequent surveillance culture results.

Management and Discussion

Although not the case for this colonized patient, invasive CRE infections necessitate aggressive and sometimes creative dosing of antimicrobial therapy as well as close clinical follow up. Most importantly, patients should undergo appropriate procedures to remove the infected source whenever possible (e.g., removal of vascular catheter, drainage of infected fluid collections).

Routine, clear communication between an acute-care hospital and surrounding LTCFs and other healthcare institutions is absolutely essential to effectively control the regional spread of antimicrobial resistance. This is especially the case for emerging pathogens such as CRE. The modern continuum of healthcare necessitates that preventive strategies be implemented in a standardized manner across a variety of healthcare settings whenever possible. Clinicians can collaborate with peers at other local institutions to promote these initiatives.

Rectal surveillance cultures for CRE can be useful to identify patients carrying these pathogens (sensitivity is >90%). According to the CDC, point prevalence testing of hospital patients for CRE carriage should be conducted following identification of CRE cases or clusters. In addition, routine active surveillance cultures might be useful for high risk populations based on local epidemiology and experience. For example, a facility might consider obtaining surveillance cultures from patients admitted from a certain LTCF(s) where CRE are known to be endemic. Alternatively, patients admitted to the intensive care unit (ICU), or patients with a specific comorbid condition or recent invasive procedure might be screened. These types of targeted surveillance strategies require an understanding of local hospital epidemiology of multidrug resistant organisms in order to effectively profile high risk patients. Patients who are known CRE carriers from prior hospitalization should be placed on contact isolation precautions upon readmission to the hospital until their current colonization status can be determined. Some experts have suggested that only three consecutive negative rectal surveillance cultures exclude ongoing colonization and others rely on a combination of negative conventional cultures as well as a negative PCR-based test. Given the serious and potentially untreatable nature of some of these pathogens, extreme caution is warranted before the decision is made to discontinue precautions for such individuals. As has been noted, the process of "flagging" patients (electronically or manually) from whom CRE or other multidrug resistant organisms (MDRO) have been isolated facilitates infection control efforts at the time of hospitalization and can decrease the transmission rate of MDROs.

Case Conclusion

This case highlights the challenges associated with managing patients who are infected or colonized with gram-negative MDROs, specifically ESBLs and CREs. Unnecessary antimicrobial therapy is unfortunately very common in hospitals and creates a "selective pressure" which promotes antimicrobial resistance, such as was the case for this patient. Clear communication between Infection Control, Infectious Diseases, and attending physician resulted in a favorable outcome in this case. The patient was not treated with antibiotics, but was placed on contact precautions until he was transferred back to the nursing home. Good communications between the tertiary care facility and his surroundings are a crucial part of infection control efforts in the era of modern continuum of medical care.

Suggested Reading

Boscia JA, Abrutyn E, Kaye D. Asymptomatic bacteruria in elderly persons: treat or do not treat. Ann Intern Med 1987;106:764–765.

Guidance for control of infections with carbapenem-resistant or carbapenemase-producing Enterobacteriaceae in acute care facilities. MMWR Morb Mortal Wkly Rep 2009; 58:256–260.

Schwaber MJ, Carmeli Y. Carbapenem-resistant Enterobacteriaceae: a potential threat. JAMA 2008;300:2911–2913.

Shlaes DM, Gerding DN, John JF Jr, Craig WA, Bornstein DL, Duncan RA, et al. Society for Healthcare Epidemiology of America and Infectious Diseases Society of America Joint Committee on the Prevention of Antimicrobial Resistance: guidelines for the prevention of antimicrobial resistance in hospitals. Clin Infect Dis 1997; 5:584–599.

Smith PW, Bennett G, Bradley S, Drinka P, Lautenbach E, Marx J, et al.; SHEA; APIC. SHEA/APIC guideline: infection prevention and control in the long-term care facility. Infect Control Hosp Epidemiol 2008;29:785–814.

Chapter 9c

Vancomycin-Resistant Enterococcus

Cassandra D. Salgado

Case Presentation

A 58-year-old woman presented to the Emergency Department complaining of headache of 3 days duration. While awaiting evaluation she suddenly vomited and became unresponsive. Emergent imaging of the brain revealed a subarachnoid hemorrhage from a left posterior communicating artery aneurysm. She underwent endovascular coiling of the aneurysm and was admitted to the neurosurgical intensive care unit. Her stay was complicated by hospital-acquired pneumonia and acute respiratory distress syndrome (ARDS) for which she received an eight day course of vancomycin and cefepime. Additionally, she had cerebral vasospasm with infarction of the left anterior and middle cerebral artery territories. This lead to hydrocephalus and she underwent ventriculoperitoneal (VP) shunt placement. She remained on the ventilator but was able to communicate. On the eleventh hospital day she developed fever of 102.7°F and altered mental status. Physical exam revealed tachycardia of 112 beats per minute, coarse breath sounds bilaterally, and right sided weakness. The exit site of an internal jugular central line appeared normal as did the VP shunt site. Complete blood count revealed a WBC count of 17.2 K per cubic MM with 82% neutrophils and 5% bands. Urinalysis revealed trace blood but was otherwise unremarkable. Cerebral spinal fluid (CSF) was obtained through the VP shunt and was hazy without xanthochromia. In the CSF RBC count was 1,755 per cubic MM, WBC count was 1,470 per cubic MM with 97% neutrophils, glucose was 8mg/dl (serum glucose 122), and protein was 233mg/dl. Gram stain of the CSF revealed numerous RBC and WBC as well as gram-positive cocci. Blood cultures (one set drawn through the central line and two sets drawn peripherally) were obtained. Chest radiography revealed stable diffuse airspace disease consistent with ARDS. She was empirically started on vancomycin and meropenem.

Differential Diagnosis and Initial Management

The differential diagnosis for this complex critically ill patient with nosocomial fever would include catheter-associated bloodstream infection, ventilator-associated pneumonia, and catheter-associated urinary tract infection; however, given her altered mental status accompanied by the abnormal CSF findings, nosocomial meningitis, ventriculitis, or periventricular abscess must be highly considered. Risk factors for nosocomial central nervous system infection include recent (within 30 days) head trauma or neurosurgery, the presence of a neurosurgical device (ventriculostomy, ventriculoperitoneal shunt, or Ommaya reservoir), and CSF leak. Given that she has been in the hospital for 11 days she is at risk for infection from nosocomial pathogens such as *Staphylococcus aureus*, Coagulase-negative staphylococci, *Enterococcus* species, Enterobacteriaceae, and *Pseudomonas* species, including antibiotic-resistant strains of these organisms. Empiric coverage with broad-spectrum antibiotics is appropriate until further workup can be done and cultures have returned.

Case Presentation (Continued)

The patient's VP shunt was removed and an external ventriculostomy was placed. Her condition did not improve significantly over the next 24 hours with continued fever. CT imaging of the brain revealed findings consistent with a ventriculitis (Fig. 9.3). Blood cultures remained negative; however, CSF cultures were positive for *Enterococcus faecium* after 48 hours and this was confirmed as vancomycin-resistant the next day. Vancomycin therapy was changed to linezolid in combination with gentamicin based on in vitro synergy data and the meropenem was discontinued after CSF cultures were finalized. Repeat CSF fluid analysis (after 72 hours of appropriate therapy) revealed WBC of 240/mm^3, with 52% neutrophils and 40% lymphocytes, RBC of 160/mm^3, glucose of 89mg/dl (serum glucose was 103), and protein of 60mg/dl.

Discussion

Enterococci are normal flora of the gastrointestinal and genitourinary tract of humans. Enterococci become resistant to vancomycin by acquisition of vancomycin resistance gene clusters, most commonly the *vanA*, *vanB*, or *vanD* genes. The product of these genes ultimately leads to the substitution of D-Ala-D-Ala-ending peptidoglycan precursors within the cell wall with D-alanyl-D-lactate termini. This altered terminus has markedly decreased affinity for binding with vancomycin, rendering the drug inactive. Vancomycin-resistant *Enterococcus* (VRE) has been reported as a cause of several different healthcare acquired infections including central line associated blood stream infections, endocarditis, catheter associated urinary tract infections, wound infections, and rarely meningitis. The vast majority of clinically relevant isolates of VRE are *E. faecium*. The incidence of VRE has been steadily increasing in US hospitals with the latest reports from the Centers for Disease Prevention and Control (CDC) stating that more than 30% of enterococci isolated from hospitalized patients are resistant to vancomycin. Risk factors for acquisition of VRE include previous receipt of antibiotics, lengthy hospitalization, particularly within an ICU, immunosuppression, the presence of a medical device (e.g., urinary catheter or central line), and close proximity to another patient with VRE.

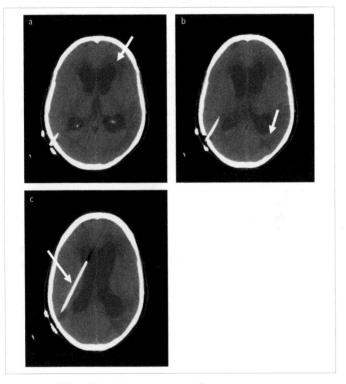

Figure 9.3 CT Scan of Brain Without Intravenous Contrast
There is hydrocephalus with prominent periventricular edema. This is highlighted by
the *arrow* in panel **A**. Isodense collections with wavy contours are described within the
occipital horns bilaterally compatible with an infectious process. This is highlighted by the
arrow in panel **B**. The ventricular shunt catheter is located within the right frontal horn.
This is highlighted by the *arrow* in panel **C**.

Much of the data regarding the impact of infection due to VRE has been
among patients with bloodstream infections wherein vancomycin-resistance
contributes to increased morbidity, mortality, and cost of care. A recent
meta-analysis of studies of patients with enterococcal bloodstream infections
reported a 2.5-fold increased risk of death (Fig. 9.4). Colonization with VRE
increases the risk of infection with studies reporting that 4% to 34% of colonized patients develop subsequent infection. Risks for developing infection
among colonized patients include infection at a distant site, residence in a long-
term care facility, and receipt of vancomycin. Treatment of infection caused
by VRE is often challenging because there are limited available antimicrobials
with activity against the organism (Table 9.3). Additionally, multidrug resistance
(most notably to synergy with the aminoglycosides) is common.
 Guidelines for control of VRE in healthcare facilities have been published and
recommend a multifaceted approach. This would include providing education

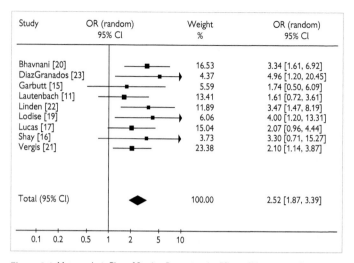

Figure 9.4 Meta-analysis Plot of Studies Reporting the Effect of Vancomycin Resistance on Mortality among Patients with Enterococcal Bloodstream Infections
The *dots* represent the point estimates for the measure of effect of each study. The *horizontal lines* represent the 95% confidence intervals for each study. The *rhomboidal figure* represents the summary measure and 95% confidence interval. The right column shows the numeric values for each study and summary measure.

(Figure used with permission from DiazGranados CA, Zimmer SM, Klein M, and Jernigan JA. Comparison of mortality associated with vancomycin-resistant and vancomycin-susceptible enterococcal bloodstream infections: a meta-analysis. Clin Infect Dis 2005;41:327–333.)

regarding the importance of the organism, use of infection prevention bundles, prudent use of antimicrobial agents, and prevention of transmission. Like other multidrug-resistant organisms, VRE is largely spread from patient to patient through the contaminated hands, clothing, and medical equipment of healthcare workers. Additionally, environmental contamination is frequent and has served as a reservoir for acquisition. Taking these factors into account, several strategies have been described to prevent transmission in the acute care setting. CDC has described this in a tiered approach. For routine control, in addition to standard precautions (which includes compliance with hand hygiene), any patient known to be colonized or infected with the organism should be placed into contact precautions (private room when available, use of a gown and gloves when caring for the patient) and noncritical medical items should be dedicated for use with these patients. Additionally, hospitals should follow the recommended cleaning, disinfection, and sterilization guidelines for maintaining patient care areas. When the incidence or prevalence of VRE is not decreasing despite the use of routine control measures or when an outbreak has been declared, intensified control efforts are needed. This could include instituting a program of active surveillance to identify colonized patients in order to fully realize the effectiveness of contact precautions, enhanced environmental cleaning and decontamination, as well as adjunctive measures such as use of topical agents for decolonization (e.g. chlorhexidine bathing).

Table 9.3 Profiles of Antibiotic Options for Vancomycin-Resistant Enterococcus faecium

Antibiotic	Mechanism of Action	Susceptible MIC (mg/L) and Antibacterial Effect	Protein Binding [%]	CSF Penetration [%]	Half-Life[b] (hours)	Adult Intravenous Doses[b]	Activity Based on in vitro Studies[c]
Chloramphenicol	Inhibits protein synthesis	≤8 Bacteriostatic	50–80%	50% with noninflamed meninges	2–4	25 mg/kg every 6 h (maximum 6 g/day)	Indifference: quinupristin/dalfopristin (combined ~80% of 28 isolates)[13,16,18], quinupristin/dalfopristin plus gentamicin or ampicillin (100% of 6 isolates)[18]
Daptomycin	Depolarizes membrane; inhibits protein, DNA, and RNA synthesis	≤4 Bactericidal	90–95%	5–6% with inflamed and 2% with noninflamed meninges[27,29,30]	7–8	6 mg/kg every 24 h (≤12 mg/kg used h this case series)	Synergy: rifampin (75% of 24 isolates were resistant to linezolid)[19,d] ampicillin (64% of 42 isolates)[12e] Indifference: gentamicin[1f]
Linezolid	Inhibits protein synthesis	≤2 Bacteriostatic		28–70%[10,14]	4–5	600 mg every 12h	Indifference: doxycycline[g]
Quinupristin/dalfopristin	Inhibit protein synthesis	≤1 Bacteriostatic	23–32%/50–56%	Poor	0.85/0.70	7.5 mg/kg every 8 h	Synergy: doxycyline (50% of 12 isolates), ampicillin/sulbactam (23% of 12 isolates), and vancomycin (17% of 12 isolates)" Indifference: ampicillin (100% of combined 16 isolates)[13,18], chloramphenicol (~80% of combined 28 isolates)[13,16,18], doxycycline (10 isolates)[13,g], gentamicin (100% of combined 19 isolates)[13,15,18] tigecycline[20], vancomycin[16] Antagonism: ofloxacin[15]

Table 9.3 Profiles of Antibiotic Options for Vancomycin-Resistant Enterococcus faecium

Antibiotic	Mechanism of Action	Susceptible MIC (mg/L) and Antibacterial Effect	Protein Binding [%]	CSF Penetration [%]	Half-Life[b] (hours)	Adult Intravenous Doses[b]	Activity Based on in vitro Studies[c]
Telavancin	Disrupts cell membrane; inhibits cell wall synthesis	≤0.29 Bactericidal	93%	2% with inflamed meninges	7–9	10 mg/kg every 24 h	Unavailable
Tigecycline	Inhibits protein synthesis via 30S subunit ribosomes	≤ 0.25 Bacteriostatic	71–89%	Undetermined	27–42	100 mg followed by 50 mg every 12h	Indifference: quinupristin/dalfopristin[20], gentamicin, vancomycin, and doxycycline[17]; rifampin (86% of combined 7 isolates)[17,20]

CSF = cerebrospinal fluid; MIC = minimum inhibitory concentration.

[a] Data obtained from product information sheets available through the Food and Drug Administration Web site (www.accessdata.fda.gov,' scripts/order/drugatfda/index.cfm).

[b] Doses and half-lives for patients with normal renal (creatinine clearance >50-60 mL/min) and hepatic functions. Dose adjustments may be necessary for patients with renal or hepatic dysfunction.

[c] Unless otherwise noted, all studies used time-kill techniques to evaluate for synergy and some in vitro studies evaluated <5 vancomycin-resistant E. faecium isolates. For combination of antibiotics when compered with the most active single agent of the combination using time-kill studies, synergy was defined as ≥ 2 log10 cfu/mL decrease in bacterial colony count, indifference as <2 log10 cfu/mL decrease in colony count and antagonism as ≥1-2 log10 cfu/mL increase in colony count.

[d] "Using E test technique in another study, 57% of 42 isolates displayed synergy when daptomycin was combined with rifampin.[12]

[e] This study used the E test technique for synergy testing.

[f] Addition of gentamicin to daptomycin increased rapidity of bactericidal activity.[11] Using the E test in a different study, 21% of isolates displayed synergy when daptomycin was combined with gentamicin.[12]

[g] In addition to time-kill studies, most strains were indifferent when combined with doxycycline using checkerboard studies (even though 36% of 50 clinical isolates displayed synergism).[13]

[h] Another study reported synergy with tigecycline and vancomycin using the checkerboard technique, but indifference using time-kill studies.[20] MIC90 for vanA and vanBtypes are 8 and 2 mg/L respectively.[21]

Used with permission from Le J, Bookstaver PB, Rudisiii CN, Hashem MG, Iqbal R, James CL, Sakoulas G. Treatment of meningitis caused by vancomycin-resistant Enterococcus faecium: high-dose and combination daptomycin therapy. Ann Pharmacother 2010;44:2001-2006.

Case Conclusion

After 14 days of appropriate antimicrobial therapy the patient had the external ventriculostomy removed and a new ventriculoperitoneal shunt placed. Antibiotics were continued another seven days (a total of 21 days of appropriate antimicrobial therapy). Over the course of the subsequent 2 weeks her condition slowly improved, she was able to be weaned from the ventilator, and was discharged to a rehabilitation center. Three additional patients in the neurosurgical intensive care unit were identified as VRE colonized and intensified control measures were adopted including a program of active surveillance, contact precautions, enhanced cleaning, and chlorhexidine baths. No additional cases of VRE infection occurred in the unit over the ensuing three months.

Suggested Reading

Carmeli Y, Eliopoulos G, Mozaffari E, Samore M. Health and economic outcomes of vancomycin-resistant enterococci. Arch Intern Med 2002;162:2223–2228.

DiazGranados CA, Zimmer SM, Klein M, and Jernigan JA. Comparison of mortality associated with vancomycin-resistant and vancomycin-susceptible enterococcal bloodstream infections: a meta-analysis. Clin Infect Dis 2005;41:327–333.

Le J, Bookstaver PB, Rudisill CN, Hashem MG, Iqbal R, James CL, et al. Treatment of meningitis caused by vancomycin-resistant *Enterococcus faecium*: High-dose and combination daptomycin therapy. Ann Pharmacother 2010;44:2001–2006.

Muto CA, Jernigan JA, Ostrowsky BE, et al. The Society for Healthcare Epidemiology of America guideline for preventing nosocomial transmission of multidrug-resistant strains of *Staphylococcus aureus* and *Enterococcus*. Infect Control Hosp Epidemiol 2003;24:362.

Olivier CN, Blake RK, Steed LL, Salgado CD. Risk of vancomycin-resistant Enterococcus bloodstream infection among patient colonized with VRE. Infect Control Hosp Epidemiol 2008;29:404–409.

Siegel JD, Rhinehart E, Jackson M, Chiarello L; Healthcare Infection Control Practices Advisory Committee. Management of multidrug-resistant organisms in healthcare settings 2006. Centers for Disease Control. Available at: www.cdc.gov/ncidod/dhqp/pdf/ar/mdroGuideline2006.pdf (accessed October 7, 2011).

Chapter 9d

Bioterrorism and Hospital Preparedness

J. Michael Kilby

Case Presentation

A 35-year-old previously healthy woman presents to your hospital emergency room complaining of 3 days of malaise, generalized myalgias, headache, and low grade fevers. Today she has become increasingly short of breath and has had small amounts of hemoptysis. She denies rhinorrhea, sinus congestion or sore throat. She lives alone and has not had exposure to children or family members with flu-like illness. She does not smoke or use illicit drugs. She works in a facility that processes letters and packages. Because of her government-related job, she has annual tuberculin skin tests, which have always been negative. She was urged by coworkers to seek medical attention because in the past week several people who work in the same warehouse with her have developed fevers, hemoptysis, and shortness of breath. She is aware that a man who worked near her died of unexplained meningitis yesterday.

On physical examination, she appears anxious and uncomfortable. Blood pressure 100/55, pulse 105, respirations 26/minute, temperature 38.1°C. The oropharynx is clear and there are no oral ulcers. There is nontender, shotty cervical adenopathy. The lung fields are clear but with dullness and decreased breath sounds at the right base. There are normal active bowel sounds, and no abdominal tenderness or organomegaly. There is no evidence of frank arthritis or muscle tenderness. There is no rash or edema. Complete blood count and basic chemistries are unremarkable. An arterial blood gas reveals pH = 7.48, $pCO_2 = 29$, $pO_2 = 89$ on room air. Chest radiograph reveals widened mediastinum and left sided pleural effusion (Fig. 9.5).

Diagnosis and Initial Management

The vast majority of healthy adults presenting with low grade fever and malaise have viral illnesses which do not require emergency management or an extensive evaluation. However, progressive dyspnea, tachypnea, and hemoptysis suggest that a more detailed history and urgent triage are indicated. In a nonsmoking adult without evidence of a chronic illness such as tuberculosis, hemoptysis and acute dyspnea are worrisome for potentially life-threatening

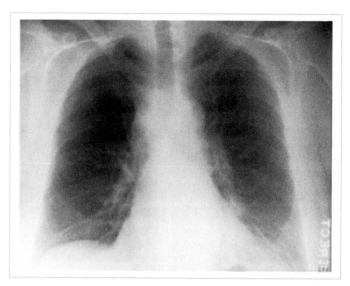

Figure 9.5 Chest radiograph showing widened mediastinum and left pleural effusion from a case of inhalational anthrax.

(Used with permission from Jernigan JA, Stephens DS, Ashford DA, at al. Bioterrorism inhalational anthrax: the first 10 cases reported in the United States. Emerg Infect Dis 2001;7:933–944)

illnesses including pulmonary embolus or bacterial pneumonia. Unfortunately, consideration of a bioterrorism event in this setting would not be likely, even with involvement of an expert Infectious Disease or Emergency Department clinician, unless there were several cases presenting concurrently or suspicions based on new media reports or government alerts.

Because you are aware of the dramatic bioterrorism events in 2001 involving anthrax sent to the offices of prominent United States federal officials, you ask for more details about the illnesses reported by her coworkers, while asking your colleagues to call her employer as well as the local and state health departments to investigate whether this possibility has been considered in your area. The occurrence of an apparent occupational outbreak involving respiratory symptoms, hemoptysis, and severe meningitis certainly parallels the 2001 experience when people who handled or opened mail were exposed to anthrax. These exposed individuals developed inhalational anthrax after a variable incubation period, typically 4 to 6 days.

Although inhalational anthrax is not spread from person to person, it seems prudent to place this patient in a negative pressure respiratory isolation room while an evaluation is under way—tuberculosis is still in the differential diagnosis and concerns about bioterrorism mean that atypical, contagious agents such as *Yersinia pestis* are at least in the realm of possibility based on suspicious events reported at her work place.

Case Presentation (continued)

Blood cultures are obtained before initiation of ampicillin/sulbactam, ciprofloxacin, and doxycycline. Sputum is obtained for Gram stain, acid fast smears, and routine cultures. A noncontrasted chest CT scan reveals mediastinal adenopathy with central hemorrhage and a large left pleural effusion. The Hospital Disaster Preparedness official on call is contacted and appropriate Centers for Disease Control officials are alerted to the evolving events. You learn that an investigation is ongoing about the events at her workplace, and that a common chemical or infectious exposure resulting from a terrorist act is a real possibility. Within 24 hours, blood cultures are growing elongated, cigar-shaped gram-positive organisms consistent with a Bacillus species (Fig. 9.6). She is admitted to the intensive care unit where she undergoes chest tube placement for worsening dyspnea, and the drainage is exudative and grossly bloody. A lumbar puncture is performed, revealing no white blood cells and a normal protein and glucose level.

Hospital Preparedness

A complete discussion about the diversity of potential bioterrorism agents is of course not possible here, but it is a useful exercise to think about the biological characteristics that a terrorist individual or organization might perceive as highest priorities: (1) HIGHLY LETHAL OR TOXIC: Inhalational anthrax may be associated with high mortality (50%–60%), although it now appears this can be

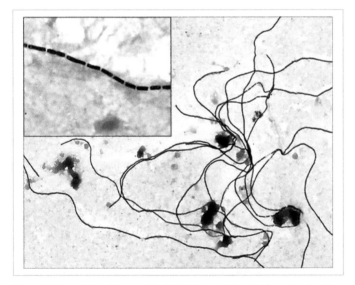

Figure 9.6 Long chains of gram positive bacilli characteristic of *Bacillus anthracis*, with segmented or beaded appearance on higher power (inset).

(Used with permission from Inglesby T, Otoole T, Henderson DA, et al. Anthrax as a biological weapon, 2002: updated recommendations for management. JAMA 2002;287:2236–2252)

markedly reduced with prompt antibiotics and hospital care. Other potential agents such as Smallpox and Viral Hemorrhagic Fevers may be associated with lesser but still substantial mortality rates (~30%). The timing of illness and death is variable with different agents—chemicals or deadly toxins such as Botulinum Toxin may act within 2 to 4 days, pneumonic plague and tularemia within a few days, inhalational anthrax within a week (but may be delayed for weeks in lower-dose exposures), whereas others such as Smallpox may have more prolonged incubation and indolent courses. (2) LIMITED OR NO PROVEN THERAPIES: Inhalational anthrax may be challenging to diagnose in a timely fashion, but therapy may be quite effective, even for severely progressive disease. Consensus guidelines suggest using multiple agents with known anthrax activity. Plague and tularemia are also quite responsive to appropriate antibiotics, but may not be adequately treated with usual empiric antibiotics for sepsis or pneumonia. Smallpox and Viral Hemorrhagic Fever viruses are examples of potentially deadly infections without proven effective therapies. (3) STABILITY AND FEASIBILITY: As proven by the U.S. anthrax attacks a decade ago, it is possible for an individual or small group with limited resources to generate sufficient anthrax for large-scale crimes. The agent of anthrax is rather ubiquitous, found in the soil in many countries for example, and can be cultured relatively easily. It forms spores that remain stable over long periods of time, also raising the possibility of creating health hazards that persist in the environment long after the initial delivery. Botulinum toxin is another example of an agent that is ubiquitous in nature and not difficult to acquire for experimentation. Smallpox is a daunting pathogen because it is stable and easily aerosolized. However, smallpox has been eradicated as a natural pathogen, and therefore the only access to it would be through a breakdown in high-security protocols at the only two sites in the world that maintain stocks for experimental purposes. Other proposed bioterrorism agents, such as *Francisella tularensis* (tularemia), retroviruses (HIV-1), or the Viral Hemorrhagic Fever viruses (Ebola, Marburg, etc.), would require a high level of sophistication and special facilities in order to prepare and deliver them, perhaps conceivable only in the setting of a heavily financed group or countrywide terrorist program. (4) INFECTIVITY: The advantage of anthrax as a deadly agent is that a small amount can be efficiently delivered via aerosolized form. The majority exposed to anthrax, especially in the developed world, would have no preexisting immunity, whether from prior exposure or immunization, so susceptibility to anthrax would be widespread in the United States. The situation is similarly ominous for smallpox because since worldwide eradication was achieved, vaccination has not been undertaken for decades and immunity is waning or absent, particularly among the youngest and healthiest of the population. Some other viruses and bacteria, even when efficiently delivered, have a variable penetrance based on complex host and pathogen factors, such that large numbers of people would have to be exposed in order to cause major casualties. Clearly, however, a major goal of bioterrorism may be to create panic and chaos, which may happen even if there only small numbers of susceptible, severely affected individuals. (5) SECONDARY SPREAD: Inhalational anthrax is generally not spread from person to person, which makes it less than ideal as an agent chosen to result in massive and ongoing casualties. It is certainly possible for exposure to skin lesions to cause additional cases of cutaneous anthrax (as occurred in a small child whose parent had been involved with processing contaminated mail in the 2001 event), but this is a cause of treatable morbidity and not frequently a cause of death. Smallpox can be spread from person to person through direct contact or airborne droplets, so that strict isolation of exposed or infected individuals in negative pressure facilities would be a high priority. Pneumonic plague also has high potential for person to person spread. While laboratory exposures to cases of tularemia or Viral Hemorrhagic Fever are a major concern, there has been little evidence to suggest that secondary spread between hosts is a common event for these agents.

Based on these principles, Table 9.4 outlines some of the highest hospital preparedness priorities for bioterrorism events.

Further Case Discussion

Anthrax can occur via inhalational, cutaneous or gastrointestinal routes, but the primary concern from the standpoint of bioterrorism is inhalational. Following a 4- to 6-day incubation period, there may only be nonspecific malaise and low-grade fever with little to suggest the possibility of a potentially deadly illness. Approximately half of patients with substantial airborne exposure may present with signs of meningitis, and meningitis due to characteristic gram positive organisms is a vital clue to distinguish what otherwise might be assumed to be a community outbreak of a viral infection. Almost all cases in the 2001 U.S. attack developed mediastinal adenopathy, although sometimes this was not appreciated on initial chest x-rays. While previous literature had suggested that pulmonary parenchymal infiltrates are not characteristic of inhalational anthrax, the majority of the 2001 victims had infiltrates or consolidation by CT scans. Most developed bloody pleural effusions requiring thoracentesis or chest tube

Table 9.4 Priorities for Bioterrorism Hospital Preparedness
A. **Designate a Coordinator** for Bioterrorism Preparedness and a multidisciplinary committee who will communicate closely with local and state health departments and the CDC.
B. **Formulate Emergency Plans**, reviewed and updated regularly, which must incorporate coverage of surrounding areas including rural locations lacking a major medical center. Close communication with microbiology experts, including those at health departments and the CDC, will be necessary to ensure access to specialized and rapid diagnostic testing.
C. Having a reasonable **Stockpile of Available Antibiotics** (including ciprofloxacin and doxycycline, as used in this example) for short-term use. The Federal Government has ramped up stockpiles tremendously, such that airliners filled with appropriate supplies (antibiotics, vaccines, etc.) can be delivered anywhere in the United States in less than 12 hours. Efforts have been made to create sufficient smallpox immunizations, for example, for the entire US population if necessary.
D. **Negative Pressure Rooms** with 6–12 air exchanges per hour (particularly relevant for smallpox or plague). If there are massive exposures, rooms typically reserved for tuberculosis care, etc., will be occupied within a short period of time. Plans will need to be considered for designating hospital wings with separate airflow or even entire buildings (schools, rehabilitation centers, etc.) as isolation areas.

management. All subjects who had blood cultures drawn prior to antibiotics were positive within 24 hours for *Bacillus anthracis*, and at least one had organisms visible on careful review of peripheral smears.

Although serologic tests and nasal cultures may be helpful epidemiologically in evaluating the extent of exposures and developing a postexposure prophylaxis plan, these results do not appear to be useful in managing the individual exposed patient. Serologic conversion requires too long to be useful for acute treatment decisions, and nasal colonization is much less definitive for proving invasive infection than demonstrating the organism in blood or CSF cultures.

A variety of antibiotics potentially have anthrax activity. A reasonable recommendation is to treat aggressively with multiple agents, to include ciprofloxacin, doxycycline, or both. Isolates should be evaluated for specific susceptibilities to assist with planning the individual and public health treatment strategy. Anthrax vaccines are available from military and CDC sources, but have been approved primarily for pre-exposure usage. Although there is the theoretical advantage of enhancing immunity to help ward off reactivation of latent spores after antibiotic treatment is completed, experiments involving nonhuman primates plus the 2001 attack experience suggest that full recovery is possible with combination antibiotic therapy alone, even for patients with severely progressive disease including meningitis.

Case Conclusion

The patient is initially managed in the intensive care unit and receives intravenous antibiotics. Although Anthrax vaccination or immunotherapeutics (immunoglobulin or monoclonal antibody preparations) via a federal program are discussed, the patient decides that she would rather not receive experimental interventions at this point. Through coordination with CDC officials her blood culture isolate is rapidly confirmed to be *Bacillus anthracis* using PCR as well as microbiologic techniques. In addition, at other hospitals, the anthrax agent is confirmed to be present in the blood of at least one other coworker as well as in the cerebrospinal fluid of the male patient who died with meningitis. CDC and regional public health officials undertake the challenging task of coordinating triage and prophylactic therapy for all others (>1,000) who may have come in contact with the airborne anthrax. The patient has complete recovery, although her pleural effusion requires complicated chest tube management for more than a month, and her antibiotics are switched to oral ciprofloxacin 500 mg twice daily and doxycycline 100 mg twice daily for 60 days.

Suggested Reading

Ingleysby T, O'Toole T, Henderson DA, et al. Anthrax as a biological weapon, 2002: updated recommendations for management. JAMA 2002;287:2236–2252.

Jernigan JA, Stephens DS, Ashford DA, et al. Bioterrorism-related inhalational anthrax: the first 10 cases reported in the United States. Emerg Infect Dis 2001;7:933–944.

Stern EJ, Uhde KB, Shadomy SV, Messonnier N. Conference report on public health and clinical guidelines for anthrax. Emerg Infect Dis 2008;14(4)pii:07–0969.

Index

"f" indicates material in footnotes and "t" indicates material in tables.

211